Thomas T. Thompson, M.D.

Chief, Radiology Service, Veterans Administration Hospital;
Assistant Professor of Radiology and Assistant Professor of Community
Health Sciences, Duke University Medical Center, Durham, North Carolina

Little, Brown and Company, Boston

Published November 1973

Primer of Clinical Radiology

Copyright © 1973 by Little, Brown and Company (Inc.)

First Edition

Library of Congress catalog card No. 73-2117

ISBN 0-316-84169

Printed in the United States of America

TO MY FAMILY, FRIENDS, AND STUDENTS

Preface

PRIMER IS DEFINED as a small introductory book on a subject. *Primer of Clinical Radiology* was written with this definition in mind. It presents an elementary understanding of radiology suitable for allied health, nursing, and medical students. Material for the book was drawn from the author's experience as a family practitioner, as a radiologist in a major medical center, and from five years of experience in developing a clinical radiology curriculum for the Physician's Assistant Program of Duke University.

The format of the clinical chapters is such that pertinent anatomy of the subject is discussed along with significant roentgenographic physiology. Clinical manifestations of familiar medical entities are then presented together with roentgenographic examples. The book covers the major portion of disease entities seen by the person delivering primary medical care to the patient.

It has not been the purpose of the author to go into detail concerning any particular subject but to try to develop a series of basic concepts on how to use roentgenographic studies for the betterment of patient care. For students who desire further information, a reference list is included. An appendix of roentgenographic bony anatomy is also included for those students who need further help in identifying bony anatomy.

I am especially indebted to my colleagues at Duke University Medical Center, who have given their valuable time in reading parts or all of the manuscript. In particular, I appreciate the help of Dr. Richard G. Lester, Professor and Chairman, Department of Radiology, who encouraged me to undertake such a monumental task; as well as the help of Drs. Charles Mansbach, A. Derwin Cooper, James T. Chen, Jack D. Davidson, Jerko Poklepovic, Robert McLelland, William F. Barry, and Mrs. Cynthia C. Kirby, RT (ARRT), of the School of Radiologic Technology, all experts in their own right.

I am also indebted to Mrs. Hazel Underwood and Mrs. Elinor Hart for assistance in the preparation of the manuscript. The illustrations were drawn by Donald G.

Powell of the Medical Illustration Service, Veterans Administration Hospital, Durham, North Carolina, and the radiographic reproductions were made on a LogEtronics reducer in the Duke-VA x-ray reproduction laboratory under the able direction of Floyd Willard, who also supervised the production of the basic positioning films.

Finally, I am indebted to Little, Brown and Company for their help and courtesies extended to me.

Thomas T. Thompson

Contents

Introduction

1

DURING THE PAST DECADE there has been a realization that in the most affluent country in the world untold numbers of people do not receive adequate medical care. The medical profession has been unable to provide adequate health care to all segments of our rapidly increasing population, primarily due to (1) lack of anticipation of the medical needs of the community, (2) inadequate funding for research, (3) insufficient construction of teaching facilities, and (4) failure to maintain competitive salaries for faculty members. Competition for qualified students from aeronautical and technological industries in the past has also resulted in the loss of many highly qualified students for medical schools.

Since World War II, mass movement of the populace to urban areas with their social and cultural advantages has contributed to a maldistribution of medical personnel. During the same period of time, a vast growth of medical knowledge has made it impossible for one person to comprehend all the current medical information. The advent of Medicare and Medicaid has opened avenues to medical care that perhaps had not existed before and also, perhaps, has opened a Pandora's box. Medical procedures are more sophisticated than before; many of today's routine clinical studies were laboratory fantasies only a few years ago.

With the demand for more medical care and the accumulation of medical knowledge and personnel in medical centers, we have entered the era of what may be termed the *doctor shortage.* There have been demands from the medical hierarchy, lay personnel, and legislative leaders that the percentage of physicians in this country be increased. Few persons realize that it costs between 50 and 100 million dollars to build a medical school and about 10 percent of the capital investment to operate it annually. A certain amount of time is required to obtain funding for such an endeavor, either through legislative action or private bequest. It takes three to four years to construct physical facilities, and an additional four years before students could be graduated. Add three to six years for specialty training, either as a family practitioner or a specialist, and

1

one has a lapse of ten years before a medical school can provide physicians for primary medical care. At least five years must be added to this to balance the loss of active practitioners from private practice who are hired by the medical center as faculty members. Therefore it takes approximately fifteen years after a medical school is conceived before any appreciable number of medical practitioners can be added to the medical profession for participation in patient care.

The following brief résumé of the delivery of medical care introduces a unique concept of furnishing such services. During the past ten years, particularly the last five years, there has been a realization by some physicians (ignored by many physicians) that some of their routine duties can be delegated to allied health workers without decreasing the quality of medical care. This concept of delivering health care was perfected by Duke University Medical Center some eight years ago. The newer members of the allied health team are known collectively as physician's associates (physician's assistants) and individually by such titles as medical assistant, patient-care technician, orthopedic assistant, child health associate, and nursing assistant.

The use of assistants is not new, however. The concept of physician's assistants dates back to the time of the Roman Empire, when "barbers" would attach themselves to armies and tend to the wounds of the soldiers. These medieval barbers, through the ages, have become the surgeons of today; the physician of ancient times would not lower himself to go on the battlefield and possibly soil himself. In later years the Russian Feldscher (field-barber) and the "Deaner" of the pathologists were utilized. The turn of the century witnessed the development of new allied health workers whom we now call *nurses.* Prior to 1930 few other allied health workers existed, and most medical care was performed by physicians. Through new developments in education, some of the duties of physicians have been relegated to those less educated but still having a high degree of skill, for example, the x-ray technician. As the complexities of medicine have increased, more and more duties have been delegated to allied health personnel, so that today there are over 200 types of such persons. The development of allied health is, in fact, the application of industrial engineering concepts to the field of medicine, designed to increase effectiveness and efficiency in the delivery of health care.

This textbook is the result of five years of teaching allied health personnel the basic principles of radiology. It is an introduction to clinical radiology and is directed toward students in physician's associate, medical, and nursing programs. The advanced radiologic technologist also may find it beneficial. The medical students who read the manuscript found it helpful as an introduction to the art of roentgenographic interpretation.

The subject matter has been chosen to reflect the great majority of the clinical entities seen in the physician's office and in a large, active radiology department. Some complex subjects such as the head and neck, congenital heart disease, bone tumors, and bony dysplasias have been purposely omitted, as through experience we have found these subjects to be inappropriate for those toward whom this textbook is directed.

The format of the subject presentation is a review of and emphasis on basic roentgen anatomy and a brief summary of the medical and radiographic findings as applied toward a disease process. The subjects are also arranged in such a fashion that the student is gradually led into an appreciation of the subtle changes shown on a radiograph and interpreted by the radiologist.

For students of radiology, this publication will appear to be an unusual undertaking. The author has attempted to develop an "understanding" of diagnostic radiology which will be useful to members of the allied health care team in their training. Information useful to only one member of the paramedical team has been eliminated, since it is believed that such is available in other radiology texts.

Most of the information contained in this text is that which is thought to be common knowledge within the medical community. The reader is referred to a selected list of readings at the end of each chapter for more detail concerning the subjects.

READING LIST

Jones, M. D. *Basic Diagnostic Radiology*. St. Louis: Mosby, 1969.

Meschan, I. *Normal Radiographic Anatomy,* 2d ed. Philadelphia: Saunders, 1959.

Meschan, I. *Roentgen Signs in Clinical Practice.* Philadelphia: Saunders, 1966.

Paul, L. W., and Juhl, J. H. *The Essentials of Roentgen Interpretation,* 3rd ed. New York: Hoeber Med. Div., Harper & Row, 1972.

Squires, L. F. *Fundamentals of Roentgenology.* Cambridge: Harvard University Press, 1964.

Storch, C. B. *Fundamental Aids in Roentgen Diagnosis.* New York: Grune & Stratton, 1951.

Sutton, D. (Ed.). *A Textbook of Radiology.* Baltimore: Williams & Wilkins, 1969.

Teplick, J. G., Haskin, M. E., and Schmidt, A. P. *Roentgenologic Diagnosis.* Philadelphia: Saunders, 1967.

Physical Foundations of Radiology

2

HISTORY OF RADIOLOGY

The important events leading to the discovery of x-rays (now called roentgen rays) are common to the fields of physics, mathematics, and electronics. The names of Gilbert, Newton, Watson, Franklin, Volta, Ampère, Ohm, Faraday, and Henry represent sources of knowledge upon which the science of radiology was built. The name of Wilhelm Konrad Roentgen should also be included in this list of distinguished investigators.

In November of 1895, Roentgen, using a Crookes's cathode ray tube which had been shielded to exclude any known source of light, passed a current through the tube and noted a black line across a piece of platinocyanide paper which lay on his workbench. Not understanding the phenomenon, Roentgen hypothesized that some mysterious ray had passed from the Crookes's tube; and he termed these *x-rays,* using the standard symbol x for the unknown. Shortly thereafter, Roentgen reported his findings in a paper entitled "A New Type of Ray," which he presented at the Physical-Medical Society of Würzburg, Germany. The findings electrified the world and later led to amusing claims such as the advertisement of "x-ray-proof" women's clothing. Roentgen ultimately received the first Nobel prize in physics, awarded in 1901.

The device used by Roentgen was a pear-shaped, gas-filled glass tube which was somewhat similar to a large, old-fashioned electric light bulb. The power was supplied by means of an induction coil which, at that time, gave a very limited source of power. Erratic output from the tube resulted due to its gaseous nature. There was no target as we commonly think of in vacuum tubes; the glass wall of the Crookes's tube, in effect, was the target.

In 1913 Dr. W. D. Coolidge of General Electric's research laboratory revealed

5

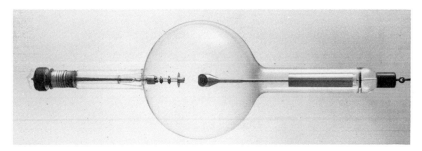

A

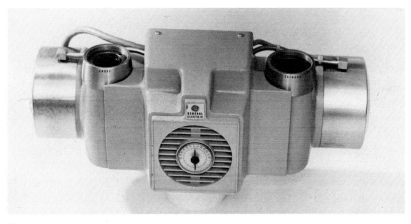

B

Fig. 2-1.
  (A) A Coolidge x-ray tube. (B) A modern General Electric Maxiray 75 x-ray tube.

the first successful "hot" cathode vacuum tube (Fig. 2-1A), which was unique if
for nothing more than its stable operation. The premise upon which this tube
was built depended upon the flow of electrons due to a voltage differential
between cathode and anode. Coolidge was also instrumental in developing a
workable tungsten alloy for use in both the cathode and anode of the new x-ray
tube. Heat dissipation from the anode became a formidable problem and ultimately led to the development of an externally activated rotating anode which
dissipated heat over a much larger surface than the stationary anode. More
efficient cooling systems were also established after the rotating anode came
into general use. With increasing needs for roentgenographic equipment over
the years, tungsten has remained the element used almost universally in cathodes,
basically because of its capability of producing large numbers of electrons and
its relatively high melting point. Recently the addition of rhenium and molyb-

denum to the target has helped to prevent melting, particularly when high-speed roentgenography is used.

In the past seventy years we have seen a rapid dissemination of roentgenographic knowledge and the development of rather markedly complicated and sophisticated roentgenographic equipment. In Roentgen's time, exposure or blackening of an x-ray film was in minutes, whereas at the present time roentgenographic exposures may be timed in milliseconds. Also in common use today are motion picture cameras which we term *cines* and television systems with videotape recorders. In some installations the use of a large-field camera similar to an aerial photography camera is a daily occurrence. In addition we have also witnessed the advance of roentgenologic techniques, nonexistent a few years ago, which aid in the diagnosis of disease processes. This is particularly true in the fields of vascular and neuroradiology, as well as in nuclear medicine.

THE PRODUCTION OF ROENTGEN RAYS

For those who have had no instruction in physics or higher mathematics, the idea of having to understand something as complicated as basic radiation physics may be alarming. It is not the purpose here, however, to teach radiation physics but only to present concepts which are applicable to radiology and which are desirable for persons performing or using roentgenographic studies to know.

In order to produce usable roentgenographic images, one must produce and control roentgen rays of varying wavelengths and direct them to a recording device so that the image can be visualized. The source of roentgen rays is an x-ray tube; and one may visualize images on roentgenographic films, fluoroscopic screens, television, or movie films.

Roentgen rays are forms of electromagnetic energy similar to visible light and radio and television signals but with shorter wavelengths. The shorter the wavelength, the more energy the x-ray wave has. Hence, the greater the energy, the better the wave will be able to penetrate matter. Longer wavelengths may be reflected from the surface of an object. Not all roentgen rays are of the same wavelength; in medical roentgenography, roentgen rays appear as a bundle, or spectrum, of energy levels or wavelengths. Roentgen rays travel at the speed of light and generally have a wavelength of 1/10,000 that of visible light.

Roentgen rays of relatively long wavelengths (relatively low energy) are useful in producing contrasty (short-latitude) x-ray films such as are required for evaluation of bone detail or iodinated contrast studies. Short-wavelength (high-energy) roentgen rays produce long-latitude films and are useful in barium studies or chest films.

The mainstay of radiology is the x-ray tube. The massive generators and transformers seen in a typical radiology suite are used to provide and control electricity for the x-ray tube. This tube is composed of an anode and a cathode enclosed in an evacuated glass container and surrounded by a lead housing. The cathode usually contains two different sizes of filaments and a focusing device which is nothing more than a hollowed-out metallic well into which the filaments are positioned. Figure 2-2 is a schematic drawing of such a tube.

Before roentgen rays are produced, electrons must be available. If one remembers some of the basic principles of physics, it will be recalled that as any element is heated, the motion of the atoms and molecules is accelerated, at some point becoming so violent that electrons are emitted from that element. In the x-ray tube, filaments composed of tightly wound tungsten wires provide the source of electrons. As the filament is heated, electrons are emitted and form a cloud around the filament. This electron cloud is focused to a small beam and is attracted to the anode of the x-ray tube by a voltage differential between the electrodes. In the x-ray tube the filaments not only must supply electrons; they must also supply a large quantity of electrons without melting. An alloy of tungsten has been developed which is not as brittle as the pure metal. This alloy is an efficient emitter of electrons, has a high melting point, and is used today in the manufacture of most x-ray tube filaments. Since one is interested in the

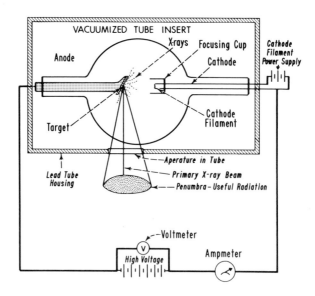

Fig. 2-2.

Basic components of an x-ray tube. Although the anode appears to be fixed, in modern x-ray tubes it rotates so as to dissipate heat over a larger surface and thus allow a greater tube capacity.

development of a large quantity of electrons from the cathode filaments, only a small amount of voltage and a large amount of amperage are applied to the filament to produce heat and subsequent motion and emission of electrons.

One can thus surmise that a large cathode filament contains more tungsten alloy than a small filament and that therefore more electrons can be produced. The resultant electron beam is also larger than that from a smaller filament and will not produce as sharp a roentgenographic image as its smaller counterpart. Unfortunately, the small filament will melt more readily than a larger one; the radiologist or radiologic technologist must take into consideration the limits and capabilities of the equipment when determining which focal spot to use for a specific procedure.

The filaments in the cathode of an x-ray tube are somewhat comparable to those in a floodlight, representing a large filament, as opposed to those in a spotlight, representing the small filament. The reflector of the floodlight or spotlight corresponds to the focusing cup of the x-ray tube. The correlation of this analogy is that if one wants detail on a roentgenograph, the smaller filament should be used (within the capability of the x-ray tube).

As with any other electron tube, the electrons are drawn from the cathode to the anode by a voltage differential applied to the anode. The amount of voltage differential determines the velocity of the electrons striking the target or anode and, hence, the quality and wavelength (energy) of the roentgen rays produced. The acceleration of the electrons is controlled by the voltage applied to the anode, and the number of electrons supplied by the cathode is controlled by the amperage applied to the filament.

The target (anode) of an x-ray tube is, like the cathode, composed of an element of high atomic weight so as to be an efficient producer of roentgen rays and yet have a high melting point because of the intense heat produced by bombardment with electrons. In earlier days, platinum was used as the target, but it has now been generally replaced by a tungsten alloy. In modern x-ray tubes, rhenium and molybdenum are even replacing tungsten as the target element. A complete vacuum must surround the anode and cathode to prevent electrons from striking gas molecules and dissipating their energy. Gas must also be removed from the metallic target for this same reason. The presence of gas will also cause oxidation of the cathode filament and completely ruin the tube.

An atom (Fig. 2-3) is composed of a nucleus surrounded by electrons in orbit. The higher the density of a substance, the closer the atoms are in relation to one another and the less motion they have. Roentgen rays result from dissipation of energy from interactions of electrons originating in the cathode as they strike the nucleus and orbitary electrons of an atom within the target of the anode. As the electrons approach the atom, two things may occur: (1) the electrons may completely miss the atom and its orbital electrons and continue through the target without dissipating any energy and hence will be absorbed by the lead

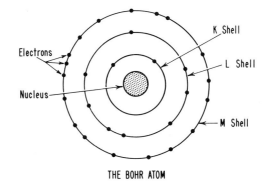

THE BOHR ATOM

Fig. 2-3.
   Bohr's atomic model with central nucleus and orbital electrons.

shielding of the x-ray tube; or (2) the electrons may interact with the nucleus or
orbital electrons of the atom and produce roentgen rays as they transfer their
energy to the atomic structure. The faster the incident electrons approach the
atomic target, the more energy will be available for conversion into roentgen
rays.

   Two types of rays are produced by interaction of the incident electrons at
the anode surface. One type is termed *characteristic roentgen rays,* and these
rays are dependent upon the atomic weight of the target element. These characteristic roentgen rays are peculiar to an element and occur when atomic electrons
change from one orbital level to another, in the process giving off energy in the
form of roentgen rays. *Bremsstrahlung* is the other type of roentgen ray produced, and it is dependent upon the energy released as the incident electron
strikes the atomic nucleus. Depending upon the energy of the incident electron,
a spectrum of energy levels is produced. Roentgen rays are emitted from the
target in all directions but are limited to the radiographic subject by a small
aperture in the lead housing of the x-ray tube. Only about 1 percent of the
energy expended into an anode target is converted into useful radiation. The
remainder of the energy is dissipated in the forms of heat and light.

   As the roentgen rays leave the radiographic tube, they strike the roentgenographic subject, and some of the roentgen rays are distorted, some are absorbed,
and some are passed directly through the subject to strike the x-ray film. Again,
those roentgen rays with higher energy levels will more readily pass through the
subject than will low-energy rays. Upon processing, the x-ray film presents an
image for viewing which corresponds to the amount of energy released and
stored permanently in the x-ray film.

   It was noted above that only about 1 percent of the energy expended in an
x-ray tube is useful in defining a roentgenographic image. In order to protect the

x-ray tube and at the same time decrease the radiation to the patient, some means must be available to enhance this radiation. This is brought about by manufacturing x-ray film to particular specifications and by the use of intensifying screens.

One of the properties of roentgen rays is the ability to cause certain material to fluoresce. Fluorescence is the capacity of a material to produce light after having been energized by light. The emitted light is of longer wavelength than the incident light. When x-ray film is manufactured, the film emulsion is produced so as to be extremely sensitive to the blue light produced by the fluorescent screens sandwiching a sheet of x-ray film. The amount of blue light produced by an intensifying screen is proportional to the amount of roentgen rays striking the screen; but since the x-ray film is so sensitive to blue light, one effectively enhances the photographic effect of the x-ray beam so that a smaller x-ray exposure is needed than would be necessary without the screen. Depending upon the character of the intensifying screen, the amount of radiation to the patient may be reduced by a factor of one-fifteenth to one-thirtieth of that normally used without an intensifying screen.

A pair of intensifying screens is mounted in a hinged metal container called a cassette. X-ray film is also manufactured with emulsion on both sides of the film. Thus each film emulsion is in contact with an intensifying screen.

Just as electrons interact with the anode of an x-ray tube to produce roentgen rays, the roentgen rays interact with body tissues to form secondary or scattered radiation. For the most part, these roentgen rays are absorbed in the body and do not contribute significantly to blackening of an x-ray film. However, when some large patients are x-rayed, scattered radiation produces a fog on the x-ray film, with a resultant decrease in film clarity. This decreased film clarity results from the scattered radiation striking the intensifying screens at other than right angles. This scattered radiation can be controlled by inserting a grid between the patient and the x-ray film. A grid is a series of thin lead strips separated by either a fiber or an aluminum spacer. Since the lead strips are perpendicular to the x-ray film, the grid has the effect of absorbing roentgen rays which will not strike the film at a right angle. Grids may be mounted in the x-ray table or directly in the x-ray film cassette.

The human body contains four definable densities: air, fat, water, and metal. The greater the density, the more radiation a material will absorb. Air, being the least dense material found in the body, does not absorb appreciable radiation and therefore allows more radiation to strike the x-ray film and intensifying screens, thus producing more film blackening upon processing of the x-ray film. At the other end of the scale, bones contain large quantities of calcium, a metal, and thus absorb more radiation, allow less film response, and produce a white image on the x-ray film. Many gradations between total black and total white occur due to the variable absorption of the x-ray beams by different tissues. The end

result is an x-ray film showing varying shades of gray which correspond to the
radiation transmitted through the body.

SPECIAL RADIOGRAPHIC PROCEDURES

We have described the basic roentgenographic process and how the roentgenographic image is produced. By varying this process, one may visualize the roentgenographic image in several different ways.

One may visualize the image directly without the aid of film by means of a
fluoroscope. This device is similar to a roentgenographic unit, but instead of the
x-ray tube being mounted above the patient, it is usually housed within the x-ray
table. As the x-ray beam penetrates the patient, it strikes a fluorescent screen
which emits a greenish yellow light as compared to the bluish light produced by
the intensifying screens. The greenish light is necessary because the human eye
is physiologically more responsive to this color. The image recorded on the
fluoroscopic screen may be enhanced to six to eight thousand times its normal
light level by means of an image intensifier. This intensified image may be
viewed indirectly by means of a mirror or by a closed-circuit television system.
If a television camera is used, video signals may then be recorded on videotape
and reviewed or analyzed at a later time. The image may also be recorded
directly on movie film; this procedure is termed *cine.*

The advantage of a fluoroscopic system is that it allows the viewer to visualize
and evaluate physiological (or pathological) motion. Unfortunately, fluoroscopic
procedures produce a large volume of radiation to the patient, some of which
may be unnecessary. Standard roentgenographs should be the examination of
choice, with fluoroscopic procedures permitted only as an alternative.

One of the more beneficial and perhaps underutilized special examinations is
that of stereoradiography. On a standard roentgenograph, three-dimensional
images are recorded on a two-dimensional film. For an experienced radiologist,
this is usually no problem. There are situations, however, which appear to occur
daily in many large radiology departments, where three-dimensional viewing is
desirable. Three-dimensional roentgenographs are produced by exposing two
roentgenographs with the x-ray tube in different positions. These roentgenographs are seen through a special viewer which allows the eyes and brain to fuse
the roentgenographs into a three-dimensional figure, thus allowing the examiner
to perceive depth.

Another commonly used roentgenographic procedure is body-section roentgenography. Several different methods are available to obtain the same goal, and
the terms *tomography, planigraphy,* and *laminography* are used interchangeably.
The goal of body-section roentgenography is to blur out images above and below
a selected body plane. By controlling the radiographic equipment, thickness of
a body section may be varied from 0.1 mm to several centimeters in width.

Tomograms are particularly useful in examining the skull (especially the mastoid areas) and bony, lung, and renal lesions.

Although this has been a superficial presentation of roentgenography, these concepts are necessary before one can appreciate and use roentgenographic procedures for the benefit of the patient.

RADIATION PROTECTION

Since the discovery of roentgen rays, there has been a fantastic growth in the use of x-ray equipment, including therapeutic units. During the past ten to twenty years, we have witnessed a rather remarkable development; and this has been especially rewarding in the areas of special procedures and nuclear medicine. There is now almost no diagnosis of a disease process which cannot in some way be aided by diagnostic radiology or nuclear medicine. It therefore behooves one to be aware of the hazards of using ionizing radiation and to become proficient in the proper use and handling of potentially dangerous diagnostic tools.

From the first atomic explosions over Hiroshima and Nagasaki, intense research has been made on the effects of radiation. Natural radiation from sources such as solar radiation, naturally occurring radioactive elements in the environment, and fallout from atomic explosions and testing gives a significant genetic radiation over which we have no control. On the other hand, the medical profession can control to some degree the level of radiation provided the patient during diagnostic and therapeutic procedures. To this end, any person who requests or uses information to be gained from roentgenographic examinations should be aware of the implications of unnecessary radiation.

The major cause of unnecessary radiation is lack of good medical judgment in ordering the studies. The responsibility for unnecessary medical radiation lies both with the person who requests the examination and with the person who performs it. This responsibility implies that one must have a sufficient knowledge of the medical implications of the various procedures. One should also question whether the same information might be available from previous studies. A large responsibility is also with the user of the equipment in that he must maintain appropriate equipment and personnel and utilize approved techniques and field sizes. It has been demonstrated, for example, that professional persons with less training in radiology than radiologists have tended to allow a primary x-ray beam which is larger than the film size, thus giving unnecessary primary and scattered radiation to the patient. Utilization of improper equipment or personnel may lead to poor diagnostic films which may necessitate repeat examination and thus repeated x-ray exposure to the patient. Fluoroscopic examinations should be limited to those areas of interest in which physiological function or motion is to be studied. For example, the chest radiograph may produce 0.5 rem radiation as compared to the 7.0 rem radiation to the patient from chest fluoroscopy.

To justify an x-ray examination, one should be certain that the information gained from the study will more than compensate for the harmful effects of radiation and that excellent, sound clinical judgment will be used in requesting an x-ray procedure.

The effects of excessive radiation are both prolonged and cumulative. Radiation affects primarily those cells which are undergoing cell division, principally found in the bone marrow and gastrointestinal mucosa, as well as in fetal and gonadal tissue. High doses of radiation produce cell death, but low doses may produce cell mutations. This is particularly important to consider when exposing gonadal and fetal tissue to low doses of radiation, as may be done in diagnostic radiology. Research has demonstrated that there is an increased incidence of cancer in patients exposed to radiation, as attested to by the increased rate of leukemia from the studies done on persons surviving the Hiroshima atomic bomb blast. There is also data to indicate an increased susceptibility to disease and a decreased life span of persons exposed to prolonged doses of radiation. This has been demonstrated by comparing the vital statistics of early radiologists to those of other persons in the medical profession. From this study it is noted that the early radiologists had a higher incidence of cancer and a decreased life span as compared to other groups of physicians. This is no longer thought to be true, since radiologists are generally aware of the hazards of radiation and tend to protect themselves. The effects of radiation are difficult to prove in man, primarily due to man's long life span; and most of the work heretofore has been done with animals.

Therefore it is incumbent upon all of us to see that damage to reproductive cells is prevented. Radiation to the gonads should be limited strictly to absolutely essential examinations, particularly during childhood, pregnancy, and the early reproductive years. Gonadal shields should be mandatory in any radiology department. Obviously it is sometimes unavoidable to include the patient's gonads within the primary x-ray beam, for example, during a barium enema or cystogram. Because of the effect on the fetus, abdominal or pelvic films on the pregnant mother are generally contraindicated. Pelvimetry should be requested only as a last resort. Radiation to the fetus should be excluded during the first trimester and allowed thereafter only in life-threatening clinical situations.

Since the effects of radiation are cumulative, the person requesting a roentgenographic examination should be aware of the amount of radiation given to the gonads in a particular examination. The books cited at the end of this chapter contain lists of the more common examinations and the relative radiation given the gonads.

READING LIST

Cahoon, J. B. *Formulating X-ray Techniques,* 7th ed. Durham, N. C.: Duke University Press, 1970.

The Fundamentals of Radiography, 10th ed. Rochester, N. Y.: Eastman Kodak Company, 1960.

Johns, H. E., and Cunningham, J. R. *The Physics of Radiology,* 3d ed. Springfield, Ill.: Thomas, 1969.

Selman, J. *The Fundamentals of X-ray and Radium Physics,* 5th ed. Springfield, Ill.: Thomas, 1972.

Radiographic Contrast Agents 3

SOME 20 TO 30 PERCENT of all radiological examinations involve the addition of a contrast medium to the body system for better visualization of that system. Contrast media are classified as pharmaceuticals by the Federal Food and Drug Administration, and thus one must have at least a fundamental knowledge of these agents in order to anticipate their effect on the patient and be able to evaluate the advisability of requesting a procedure which may involve the administration of such media. The literature contains many references concerning contrast media, but it is the purpose of this text to present the basic facts about common contrast materials in a concise form. A fairly inclusive brochure describing and classifying contrast material has been published by the Eastman Kodak Company, and the *Physicians' Desk Reference for Radiology and Nuclear Medicine* is relatively comprehensive. The reader is referred to these publications for more detailed information.

In radiology, *contrast* means "density difference." Contrast materials are "contrast" materials in the true sense of the word. The word *dye* is a poor term and a holdover from earlier days, stemming from the use of a dye, phenolphthalein, which was tagged with iodine and used in examination of the gallbladder.

Two classes of contrast material are used in radiological examinations, radiopaques and radionuclides. Radiopaques are those materials which absorb radiation; radionuclides are those which emit radiation. Air, nitrous oxide, and carbon dioxide neither absorb nor emit appreciable amounts of radiation, but they are still considered contrast materials since they produce a density difference. Radionuclides belong within the realm of nuclear medicine and will be discussed in Chapter 12. Radiopaques are divided into soluble and insoluble materials. About the only insoluble material used in radiology is barium sulfate. All the other contrast materials are soluble and contain iodine of one form or another. The commonly used contrast materials are listed in Table 3-1.

Iodine is used in soluble contrast materials basically because of its availability,

Table 3-1.

Common Contrast Materials and Their Uses

Biliary System	*Myelography*
Telepaque (iopanoic acid)	Pantopaque (iophendylate)
Oragrafin Calcium (ipodate calcium)	Air
Oragrafin Sodium (ipodate sodium)	Ascending Lipiodol (iodized oil, U.S.P.)
Cholografin (meglumine iodipamide)	Lipiodol Descendant (iodized oil, U.S.P.)
Cardiovascular System	*Pulmonary*
Same as for Urinary Tract, below.	Dionosil (propyliodone)
Generally use high concentrations;	Dionosil Oily
e.g., Renografin-76 rather than	*Sialography*
Renografin-60.	Pantopaque (iophendylate)
Gastrointestinal System	Ethiodol (ethiodized oil)
Barium sulfate, U.S.P.	Lipiodol (iodized oil)
Gastrografin (oral meglumine diatrizoate)	*Urinary Tract*
Oral Hypaque (oral sodium diatrizoate)	Renografin (diatrizoate)
Hysterosalpinography	Hypaque (diatrizoate)
Lipiodol	Conray (iothalamate)
Salpix	
Lymphangiography	
Ethiodol	

atomic number (non-metallic series), and ready exchangeability with other ions. The principal action of the contrast material depends upon the vehicle upon which the iodine is tagged. Differences in the contrast material can cause significant changes in radio-density of tissue substances and are generally related to the amount of iodine in the compound. In the United States, only two common contrast materials are used, namely, diatrizoates and iothalamates. Of these, methylglucamine and sodium salts of each are available.

It has been reported that methylglucamine salts are less toxic than sodium salts of diatrizoate or iothalamate. Viscosity is generally not a problem with contrast materials, but 90 percent methylglucamine salts of diatrizoate or iothalamate may require preheating and power injection.

The effects of contrast material upon the body are varied. All intravascular contrast materials are hyperosmotic, causing an increase in the intravascular blood volume followed by an osmotic diuresis. This can be quite deleterious, particularly in dehydrated elderly and infant patients. It has been reported that silver nitrate stains show a distinct disturbance of the endothelial lining of the blood vessels following intraarterial injection of contrast material. Contrast material also may cause crenation of blood cells and diffusion errors of cell membranes and can even affect coagulation, principally by the effect of contrast material upon fibrinogen.

Most iodinated contrast materials are excreted unchanged, either by the liver or kidneys. Maximum dosage is generally considered to be 2 to 3 ml per kilogram of body weight for intravenous or intraarterial roentgenographic studies.

Particular information concerning excretion of the contrast material is discussed below.

Inherent in the use of radiological contrast material is the ever-present distinct possibility of an adverse reaction. Concomitant with the rapid rise in the radiological subspecialties, particularly that of vascular radiology, has been the development of more ideal contrast materials; and those presently used in radiology are considered to be within safe ranges. The use of contrast materials plays a major role in diagnostic procedures, and the information to be gained by such studies generally outweighs the morbidity and slight mortality resulting from the use of contrast materials. This is due to the decreased toxicity and increased formulation of new compounds over the past ten to fifteen years. The ideal contrast material has yet to be developed, however, and it cannot be overemphasized that a death during a *diagnostic* procedure is far more significant than one occurring during a *therapeutic* procedure.

One should always be aware of the potential dangers of contrast materials, although reactions are usually relatively minor and infrequent. It is because they do occur and may happen with fatal consequences that one should always be aware of the possibilities and be fully trained to recognize such reactions and to initiate good emergency treatment. These substances are not innocuous, and safeguards should always be available.

THE SELECTION OF CONTRAST AGENTS

Biliary System. Telepaque (iopanoic acid) is given in the form of 0.5 gm tablets administered the night before the examination. Six tablets are given, one at a time, with a small drink of water. Preparation includes a fatty meal for lunch the day before the examination, a fat-free meal the night before, and usually fasting after midnight, although the patient may have clear fluids which do not contain fat.

Another oral cholecystographic agent is Oragrafin (sodium or calcium ipodate). Sodium Oragrafin is absorbed slowly and gives visualization about four hours after the drug has been ingested. Calcium Oragrafin is absorbed quickly, and the bile ducts may be seen as early as twenty minutes after ingestion of the compound; the gallbladder usually is seen about twelve hours later. Knowing that calcium Oragrafin is quickly absorbed may help one perform a gallbladder series with no patient preparation.

Visualization of the gallbladder with Telepaque depends upon its conjugation with glucuronide in the liver, the flow of the bile into the gallbladder, and the concentrating ability of the gallbladder mucosa. If the gallbladder is unable to concentrate the compound, there will be essentially no visualization. The action of Oragrafin is different in that visualization of the gallbladder by the use of this material depends upon rapid absorption from the bowel and thus an increased amount of contrast media in the biliary system, which gives more density. This may permit visualization of the gallbladder even in the presence of gallbladder disease. Therefore, nonvisualization of the gallbladder with both Telepaque and Oragrafin indicates obstruction of the cystic duct, provided liver functions are normal. Nonvisualization of the gallbladder with Telepaque does not preclude a patent cystic duct system. When the gallbladder is stimulated to contract, the contrast material occasionally may be seen faintly within the bile ducts.

If the gallbladder does not visualize with either Telepaque or Oragrafin, an intravenous compound may be used, the most common of which is a methylglucamine salt of iodipamide (Cholografin). The action of Cholografin is the same as that of Oragrafin, but there is less enterohepatic circulation. If the gallbladder has not been demonstrated on the oral study, particularly with Oragrafin, there is only a slight chance that it will visualize with Cholografin. One must remember that if the serum bilirubin is over the level of approximately 3 mg per 100 ml, the possibility of visualization with any intravenous or oral compound is highly remote and an examination would not usually be indicated.

The drugs used for the biliary system are excreted and secreted through the biliary system into the gallbladder and thence into the feces. A small amount is also excreted by the kidneys, and one may see a faint nephrogram or calyceal effect when using intravenous cholangiographic materials.

With *increasing* value of serum bilirubin and serum alkaline phosphatase, a percutaneous puncture of the biliary system can be obtained and contrast material substituted for bile. Such soluble contrast materials as Hypaque, Renografin, and Conray are used for this type of procedure. If the serum bilirubin is decreasing in value, it is generally safer to wait and do an oral or intravenous study.

Gastrointestinal System. The mainstay of examination of the gastrointestinal tract is barium sulfate, U.S.P. Barium has been pulverized, micronized, suspended, colloided, beaten, concentrated, diluted, and whatnot, but the result is still barium sulfate, with different coating characteristics and viscosity. Barium is an insoluble opaque powder usually flavored with some type of syrup for more palatability. It is of high atomic weight, producing increased absorption of the x-ray beam which, in turn, produces a white image on the radiographic film.

Barium sulfate can be used with impunity if it is used correctly. It is standard procedure not to use barium when there is a chance of communication between the bowel and the peritoneal space or the pleural space. The reasons are quite obvious, since free barium in the pleural or peritoneal space cannot be removed by physiological processes and will remain there until removed surgically. Barium by itself is essentially inert; but barium mixed with fecal material produces a severe peritonitis and granuloma formation. Not only does the barium-fecal mixture produce adverse effects; also the surgeon does not cherish the thought of operating in a field full of barium. Another restriction on the use of barium is that if barium is given orally, free passage throughout the large bowel must be possible. If barium is permitted to remain, particularly in the right colon, and if water is absorbed from it, the barium forms a rather hard fecal impaction which may have to be removed surgically.

Water-soluble compounds are used to examine the gastrointestinal tract when the presence of barium within the gastrointestinal tract may be deleterious to the patient, when there is a possibility of occlusion of the colon, or when surgery is anticipated in the near future. The principal contrast materials are compounds of methylglucamine or sodium salts of diatrizoate. The atomic weight of the iodine-containing or soluble compounds does not give as good a radiodensity as the higher atomic weight of barium. In addition, as the oral soluble compound passes through the small bowel it is diluted with succus entericus (small bowel juice), creating an even fainter image on the radiograph. Soluble compounds also create an osmotic load to the bowel, accentuating dehydration. The soluble compounds can be used for enemas, but this is relatively expensive due to the large amounts required and may cause dehydration, particularly in infants.

The use of carbon dioxide or air as a double-contrast material with barium is common in all radiology departments. This affords no pharmacological problem.

Myelography. The first contrast material used in examination of the spinal column was air, recorded by Dandy in 1918 during his evaluation and development of pneumoencephalography and ventriculography. There is no appreciable pharmacological effect of air, and the physiology concerning replacement of the spinal fluid with air is beyond the scope of this presentation. Air emboli are always a hazard. The one compound used almost universally is Pantopaque (iophendylate injection, U.S.P.), which is very slowly absorbed from the central nervous system, with the amount of absorption being equal to approximately 1 ml per year. The compound should be removed as completely as possible from the spinal column after completion of the examination, although this is open to discussion, for in some countries none is removed. Some of the side effects of the drug include headache, backache, and transient elevation in temperature, all of which are thought to be due to the lumbar puncture rather than to the drug itself. Water-soluble contrast materials generally are not used in myelography in this country because of the possibility of creating an adhesive arachnoiditis.

Bronchial Tree. Nature has provided two excellent contrast materials within the human body for examination of the bronchial tree. These are the soft tissue fluids around the bronchi, the blood vessels, and the inherent air from the environment which is distributed throughout the bronchial tree. A good contrast is made roentgenographically between the fluid and air with just the use of high-kilovoltage films. Using air as a contrast agent for planigraphy often provides one of the better examinations of the lung.

The positive contrast examination of the bronchial tree, particularly in association with bronchial brush technique and bronchial washings, is becoming a mainstay in diagnosis of pulmonary tree pathology. The agents commonly used in positive contrast examinations are heavily saturated and iodinized oils. One of the most commonly used contrast agents is Dionosil, which does not liberate free iodine and thus may be used in the presence of tuberculosis and known sensitivity to iodine. Dionosil (oily) is hydrolized and eventually coughed up, swallowed, and excreted with the feces or through the kidneys. A small portion of the contrast material is phagocytized. There does not appear to be any delayed clinical reaction or tissue damage from the use of Dionosil (oily) for bronchography.

Bronchography may not be indicated in patients with severe airway disease associated with abnormal pulmonary function. Some radiologists prefer to examine only one lung at a time, particularly in view of abnormal pulmonary function tests.

Genitourinary Tract. Roentgenographic examination of the kidneys, ureters, and bladder is routine for evaluation of fever of unknown origin, infection of the urinary tract, tumors, and anomalies. Using suitable film technique, the roentgenographic examination can also be used in evaluation of renovascular hypertension, which perhaps is one of its more common uses today.

Three commonly used drugs are Hypaque (sodium diatrizoate), Renografin (meglumine diatrizoate), and Conray (meglumine iothalamate). All may be given intramuscularly, intravenously, or intraarterially, but most commonly intravenously. Dosages as listed by the pharmaceutical companies are usually 20 to 25 ml of the regular compound (i.e., Hypaque, Renografin-60, or Conray). This is usually given slowly, as recommended by the pharmaceutical companies. However, it is a common clinical practice to use a double dose (50 to 60 ml) of the above drugs for routine urograms, with films taken at specified intervals. The use of large dosages of contrast material has a distinct advantage in that better visualization of the kidneys, ureters, and bladder can be obtained; less notice may be paid to the hydrated state of the patient; and the perpetual problem of bowel preparation is somewhat alleviated.

Good visualization of the kidneys is provided with a standard intravenous dose if the patient has been properly prepared. However, if the blood urea nitrogen (BUN) is above 25 mg per milliliter of serum, the possibility of good visualization of the kidneys usually is not likely; one must therefore consider using the drip infusion technique, which generally shows the kidneys even with the BUN as high as 100 to 110 mg per 100 ml.

The drip infusion technique for the average adult consists of the use of 150 ml of contrast material diluted with 150 ml of 5% dextrose and water. The mixture is given intravenously, either by a straight gravity drip or by the use of an intravenous "push," which is provided by using a 30 or 50 ml syringe connected through a three-way stopcock directly to the venipuncture site and to the drip infusion setup. There is now on the market a kit for drip infusion which includes premixed drugs, tubing, and a needle. Using the drip infusion technique, films are usually obtained about 2 minutes after the compound has been injected and approximately 10 minutes later. Use of the drip infusion technique further accentuates the advantages of larger doses of contrast material and quite frequently obviates the need for a retrograde pyelogram.

The actions of the different contrast materials are essentially the same. There is some variance in the viscosity of the material, which creates a problem when the contrast material is allowed to stand in a glass syringe for a short period of time. This viscosity problem is more common with the methylglucamine salt drugs than with the sodium salts. The contrast material is rapidly disseminated throughout the body and rapidly excreted unchanged through the kidneys, primarily by glomerular filtration. The contrast material has an osmotic diuretic effect which can be quite harmful, particularly in dehydrated elderly and infant patients.

The side effects of injection of contrast material include nausea, vomiting, pallor, and urticaria, with the spectrum extending as far as pulmonary edema and cardiovascular collapse. Slow injection of the contrast material is usually accompanied by few or no side effects; however, the rapid injection of contrast material is almost always attended by their increased incidence. This is almost routinely seen in the minute-sequence urogram, in which the contrast material is injected as rapidly as possible. The same side effects occur when the drip infusion technique is used and the contrast is pushed by a syringe. Some of the nausea can be alleviated by the adding of antihistamines to the compound or injecting them intravenously shortly before the injection of the contrast material.

A disadvantage of giving large volumes of contrast material is that the renal calyces, infundibulae, and pelves may be distended by the large osmotic diuretic load to the kidneys, obscuring small tumors or other pathological conditions in the same manner in which a retrograde pyelogram does. Statistically this does not appear to be an insurmountable problem.

By the use of the drip infusion technique, there is usually sufficient contrast material within the bladder to afford adequate visualization of the bladder for a cystogram. In some departments a routine voiding cystourethrogram is obtained, as there is usually enough contrast material within the bladder for adequate visualization.

The contraindications to roentgenographic examination of the urinary tract consist of previous reaction to the contrast material, multiple myeloma (if the patient is dehydrated), poor renal function with the BUN generally above 100 to 110 mg per 100 ml, hypothyroidism, and hyperthyroidism. Examinations can be performed on patients with a previous history of adverse reaction to the contrast material provided the information to be obtained from the study is more advantageous than not doing the study at all. In these cases, the patient is usually premedicated with some type of antihistamine and corticosteroids. Even in patients with multiple myeloma, an intravenous pyelogram may be performed if the patient is adequately overhydrated to prevent the precipitation of urinary protein within the kidneys and ureters. A drip infusion pyelogram should be done with caution on a patient with congestive heart failure, as the osmotic load to the vascular tree may throw the patient deeper into heart failure and, probably, pulmonary edema.

Radionuclide studies, particularly those using iodine, should always be obtained before the use of water-soluble contrast materials, as the iodine within the contrast material would negate any valid radionuclide studies of the thyroid gland. It should be remembered that any iodine-containing positive contrast material, including that used for bronchograms, myelograms, gallbladder examinations, and intravenous pyelograms will negate accurate evaluation of thyroid function for long periods of time due to the slow breakdown and release of the iodine attached to the contrast media.

Vascular Radiology. Contrast materials used in this area of radiology are essentially the same as those used in excretory pyelography, although the iodine content may be higher than in drugs used for pyelography. The greater amount of iodine affords better visualization of small venules and arterioles which, in turn, enhances interpretation of the roentgenograms. With the higher iodine content, the viscosity of the contrast material also increases, making it almost mandatory to use a power injector when injecting large quantities of contrast material over a short period of time.

Sialography. Pantopaque is one of the commonly used drugs in roentgenography of the salivary ducts. It is instilled within the excretory ducts of the salivary glands through a blunt needle or catheter, and appropriate roentgenograms are exposed. The drug can be removed by the use of lemon or other sour juice placed within the mouth, which increases the flow of saliva from the salivary glands. This, in turn, expels the contrast material from the salivary ductules. Water-soluble contrast material is usually not used in sialography due to the possibility of adhesive fibrous changes which could obscure and obliterate the ducts or ductules.

Hysterosalpinography. Examination of the uterus and oviducts is accomplished by instilling contrast material through the cervix. This then flows through the body of the uterus and thence into the oviducts. It eventually spills into the abdomen, giving visualization of the oviducts and body of the uterus. Spillage is normal in nonpathological conditions and may be accompanied by abdominal cramping, sometimes with fever and chills. Water-soluble and oil-base compounds are generally used, with the oily compounds favored by some because of a tendency for the water-soluble compounds to create adhesions and possible obliteration of the oviduct lumen. This is not particularly true of one of the newer water-soluble drugs (Salpix). Contraindications to hysterosalpinography include pregnancy and moderate to severe infection. The examination is usually performed during midportion of the menstrual cycle.

Lymphangiography. The lymph channels are identified before cannulation by the injection of small aliquots of Evans blue or patent blue violet dye between the webs of the first three toes or fingers. The dye is then picked up by the lymph and concentrated within the lymph channels, affording easy visualization. The lymph channels are then cannulated with a No. 27 or No. 30 needle, and oily contrast material (Ethiodol) is injected slowly under pressure. The contrast material flows in the lymph channels to the lymph nodes, where the material is then filtered as a foreign body, with overflow shunted to the next node, and so on. When the contrast material reaches the cisterna chyli, it is poured into the thoracic duct which eventually empties into the jugular vein; and the contrast material is then cast as microemboli into the pulmonary artery segments. These microemboli may be quite evident upon taking chest roentgenograms the day following the lymphangiogram. One criterion of lymphangiography is that the patient have adequate pulmonary function. This sometimes entails pulmonary function testing for proper evaluation, with the minimum acceptable level being 70 percent of normal. One absolute contraindication to lymphangiography is a history of irradiation of the lung fields. Care must be taken that the contrast material is injected into the lymph channels, since veins may also pick up the dye and masquerade as lymph channels. Dosage of contrast material varies according to the size of the patient but in our experience is usually approximately 7 ml for a lower extremity lymphangiogram.

Reactions to contrast material for lymphangiography are the same as those to other iodine-containing compounds, although they are less common. Extravasation of the oil into the soft tissues may sometimes create oil granulomas. One of the most frequent complications of lymphangiography is infection at the injection site. Only adequate sterile technique can prevent this complication. Lymphangiographic material within the lymph nodes may cause an inflammatory reaction with scarring of the nodes.

Other Body Systems. There are several other uses of contrast material in radiology which do not warrant separate titles. The injection of fistulas or sinus tracts is an everyday procedure and is usually accomplished with the use of water-soluble compounds (Hypaque, for example). Retrograde urethrograms may also be performed with the same drug. Injection of the canaliculi of the tear ducts may also demonstrate the tear ducts, tear sacs, and nasolacrimal ducts. Pantopaque is also used for positive contrast studies of the posterior fossa and for ventriculography.

REACTIONS TO CONTRAST MEDIA

One of the major problems in determining adverse reactions to contrast material
has been the lack of adequate reporting and follow-up of reactions to drugs.
There are essentially three different types of reactions to contrast materials. The
first is the true allergic reaction in which a protein-hapten response has occurred.
Second are those of idiosyncrasies such as the anaphylactoid reaction to the drug
in which there is no history of previous exposure. Chemotoxic reactions are the
third type.

The term *adverse reaction* is generally used rather than *drug allergy* because
there is not a single instance of demonstrated antibody against contrast material
to be found in the literature. The adverse reactions to injectable contrast material do not appear to be antigen-antibody reactions, and it has been suggested
that the effects are more closely related to hypertoxicity and contrast-protein
interaction. It is also believed that the primary biochemical change in the human
body as a response to the injectable contrast material is the massive release of
histamines, with or without a previous history of an allergic reaction.

The Significance of the Allergic History. Before even considering the injection of
contrast material into the human patient, one must always question the patient
concerning the presence of an allergic history, particularly since it has been noted
that the instance of adverse reactions is more likely to occur in patients who have
an allergic history. This fundamental rule should be remembered: *ALWAYS
ASK THE PATIENT IF HE HAS AN ALLERGIC HISTORY AND, IF SO, TO
WHAT DRUGS OR FOODS.* One of the most common allergic reactions is that
to penicillin, followed closely by reactions to sulfa drugs. The patient should be
questioned about any previous injection of contrast material and whether there
was an adverse reaction at that time. It should be remembered that it is quite
common to have minor adverse reactions such as flushing, tachycardia, and
nausea and vomiting that may be the effect of the hyperosmality of the drug
rather than a true adverse reaction. Note should also be made of the possibility
of precipitation of protein within the renal tubules in patients having multiple
myeloma. The chance that large doses of contrast material given to patients
with suspected pheochromocytoma can cause a very dramatic rise in the systolic
blood pressure should also be remembered.

The allied health worker should always be in the habit of routinely looking at
the label of any drug to be certain that the drug is what it is supposed to be and
contains the proper percentage of iodine. It should also be noted that there is an
"average" dose which must be individualized according to the size of the patient.
Injection of radiopaque contrast material should be done only by those who are
properly trained, but occasions may arise in which the student might inject such
materials. Before any injection is made, certain drugs should be available,
namely, Benadryl in a 50 mg vial and Adrenalin, 1:1,000 (take 0.1 or 0.2 ml

and dilute to 1 ml with sterile saline and label); Solu-Cortef in a ready-mixed vial should also be available. Emergency equipment and drugs should always be readily available before any contrast material is ever injected.

Medicolegally, a test dose must be given to every patient. As has been shown time and time again, this is not an indication of whether the patient will have an adverse reaction to the contrast material, but, because of our legal responsibility, it must be done. The quickest way to give the test examination is to inject 0.2 to 0.5 ml of the substance intravenously and then wait 1 to 2 minutes with the needle in place before the rest of the contrast material is injected. After the injection has been made, the allied health worker should be readily available for 5 minutes in the same area and generally available for the next 30 to 60 minutes. Although most reactions occur within the first 5 minutes after injection of the contrast, it is not uncommon for a reaction to occur some time later than this.

There is a controversy as to the advisability of routinely injecting antihistamines before the administration of contrast material. Some physicians believe that prior injections of antihistamines will mask a minor reaction and are thus inadvisable; whereas others believe that treatment of a reaction should be done before the reaction is manifest.

The Mild Reaction. Mild reactions to contrast material include nausea, vomiting, hives, and urticaria. It is important to recognize that the rapid injection of contrast material intravenously (for example, during rapid-sequence urography) will make many patients nauseated, and this is not considered an adverse reaction but merely a side effect of the drug. It is generally uncommon for a significant drug reaction to be accompanied by nausea and vomiting; these side effects are considered to be secondary to the hypertonicity of the contrast material. Nevertheless, intravenous — never intramuscular — injection of an antihistamine (Benadryl, 10 to 15 mg, or Dimetane, 10 mg) will quickly counteract such a side effect, primarily due to the antiemetic effect of antihistaminic drugs. Some authors also question the advisability of giving antihistamines even to treat the nausea occurring from the drug injection. It is significant to realize that any mild reaction may be followed by a severe one. The injection of steroids or Adrenalin is never indicated for this mild type of reaction.

The second most severe reaction is that of urticaria, or hives. Hives are generally identified by single or multiple widespread millimeter-to-centimeter-sized punctate, erythematous lesions. Occasionally only one will appear, but it is quite common to see them scattered over the entire body. Urticaria may present as a redness around the neck or face, followed by severe itching of the entire body. Hives and urticaria are important in that they may be the forerunner of a more severe reaction such as respiratory distress or cardiac arrest or both. Immediately upon the appearance of hives or urticaria, the patient should be given an antihistaminic, preferably Benadryl or Dimetane, intravenously in the *opposite* arm or extremity from that in which the infusion of contrast material was made. If another vessel is not readily available and if a venipuncture is still present, that site may be flushed with sterile saline and the injection made in that site. It should be noted that some antihistamines, particularly Benadryl, will create a precipitate with the contrast material; and care must be taken that such a precipitate is not injected into the patient.

The intravenous injection of an antihistaminic will almost always counteract the hives and urticaria quickly, usually within 2 to 3 minutes. The patient must be watched closely and must have his blood pressure monitored and his chest examined with a stethoscope to be certain there are no cardiac arrhythmias or respiratory wheezings. If the antihistaminic does not counteract the appearance of the hives or if the urticaria increases, the patient should be given Adrenalin intravenously (1:1,000, 0.2 ml diluted to 1.0 ml with sterile saline and slowly titrated), giving only 0.1 or 0.2 ml of the *diluted* Adrenalin mixture.

Even though hives or urticaria are usually minor allergic reactions, an intravenous administration of sterile saline, 0.9%, or 5% dextrose in water should be given by the drip infusion method. All pillows should be removed from under the patient's head, and he should be made as warm and comfortable as possible. A physician should be notified immediately of the possibility of a severe allergic reaction. It is not necessary to monitor the patient's blood pressure, as one will come to know with experience that a full-pounding pulse indicates that no blood pressure drop has occurred. However, it is necessary to make certain that the patient does not develop respiratory wheezing. Also, the *patient's physician,* as well as the radiologist, should be notified of the occurrence of a reaction to contrast media, since it is always possible to have a delayed reaction from one to two hours after the patient has left the radiology department. It is generally accepted that the intravenous solutions may be safely removed when all hives have disappeared and the patient no longer has urticaria. If the patient's hives or urticaria are still present but the patient is otherwise asymptomatic and has stable vital signs, he may be sent directly to the ward to be under his own doctor's supervision. This should always be done at the direction of the radiologist.

The Severe Reaction. Severe reactions may occur without warning, but a good indication of the possibility of an acute reaction is extreme anxiety on the part of the patient. During these occasions, the blood pressure and pulse must be monitored closely. If there is any change in pulse rate or blood pressure, the patient should immediately have his head lowered to the table top and be made as warm and comfortable as possible. Immediately upon the appearance of any respiratory wheezing, the patient's neck should be hyperextended to maintain the all-important adequate airway. If the patient's heart rate continues to be normal and there is no change in blood pressure, intravenous administration of fluid such as saline or 5% dextrose in water should be started. The radiologist should be informed immediately of such a reaction. Depending upon the arrangements made by the radiologist, an anesthesiologist should also be notified. The sequence of administration of drugs is the same as noted above in that Benadryl or some type of antihistaminic should be administered intravenously. If the respiratory wheezing still continues, the antihistaminic should be followed within 2 to 3 minutes by intravenous Adrenalin mixed as stated above. Quite often the patient must be given Solu-Cortef, which should be readily available in a ready-mixed vial for administration in only a few seconds. The entire vial of 250 mg is mixed and injected slowly intravenously. At this moment the patient's life is literally in the hands of the person treating him. If respiratory or cardiac arrest occurs and no physician is available, the allied health worker must make an all-out effort to sustain life until indications for stopping such procedures are given by a physician.

The Management of Cardiac Arrest. The first few seconds are the most valuable time the patient has. During this period, the paramedic must react if the patient's life is to be sustained. The brain is the most valuable organ and the most vulnerable to lack of oxygen. It may be damaged irreversibly by anoxia, which occurs if oxygen is lacking for as short a time as 4 minutes. There are certain exceptions to this rule, such as hypothermia, which are beyond the scope of this presentation.

The first reaction of the person discovering an absence of vital signs should be an immediate call for assistance. He should then look quickly for obvious upper airway obstruction and then begin mouth-to-mouth resuscitation and closed cardiac massage.

The second person to arrive should immediately begin external cardiac massage. It is presumed that the patient is most likely on an x-ray table, which serves as an excellent chest board. As soon as possible, a plastic airway should be inserted and respiration continued with the use of a self-inflating bag such as an Ambu bag.

If a venipuncture has not been performed, this should be done by the next person to arrive. It must be remembered that the intravenous catheter should be of sufficient size to force fluid. A No. 21 scalp vein needle is not acceptable. Since paramedical personnel act as agents of a physician, it is strongly believed that no further administration of drugs should be made without the direct order of a physician. The resuscitation team should be aware of the location of all emergency equipment within the department, including emergency drugs and means of administration.

Some basic factors should be pointed out in the management of cardiac arrest. An open airway is the most important element for treatment of cardiac arrest. It is a rare patient who cannot have an adequate airway established simply by hyperextending the neck and pulling the jaw forward. Obviously the mouth should be explored to remove dentures or any other foreign body or vomitus. A plastic airway should be inserted to hold the tongue forward and facilitate suction and ventilation with an Ambu bag. Management of anoxia is extremely important due to some fundamental observations: (1) anoxia that develops during resuscitation is just as damaging as the initial anoxia without ventilation. (2) The development of anoxia further hinders the treatment of ventricular fibrillation or other cardiac arrhythmia if the heart is hypoxic. If external cardiac defibrillation is performed, the patient should be hyperventilated just before the external shock is applied and hyperventilated immediately after the procedure.

In order to perform mouth-to-mouth ventilation, the operator should be in a comfortable position at the side or slightly above the shoulder level of the patient. One hand is placed behind the neck to hyperextend the neck and hold the jaw forward. The nostrils are pinched shut with the other hand, and the operator exhales forcibly and directly into the patient's mouth about 15 times per minute. If a plastic airway is available, this can be substituted for direct mouth-to-mouth contact. Proof of good ventilation is visible expansion of the chest. It should be standard in any radiology department that a free-breathing, self-inflating bag is always available, for example, the Ambu bag. These free-breathing bags have a connection for attachment to an oxygen source, and this type of ventilation should be substituted as soon as possible for mouth-to-mouth breathing. If oxygen is available, the flow rate should be approximately 15 meters per minute. If the operator is so experienced, an endotracheal tube should be inserted with direct laryngoscopy, as this provides a direct route to the lungs, facilitates suctioning, and decreases the likelihood of aspiration. Intubation also permits the use of a mechanical respirator and is a nearly ideal way to overcome mechanical problems of ventilation, including dead space. Endotracheal intubation should not be attempted by the inexperienced, as the time lapse will create a severe anoxia which may cause brain damage. At this time, a physician should be available for further guidance.

It has been established that external cardiac compression is an effective way to restore cardiac output. It is well to remember some of the basic points in external cardiac massage, outlined below.

1. The patient's chest should be on a firm surface; and it is presumed that in treatment of allergic reactions to contrast material the patient will be on an x-ray table, which serves as an adequate, firm surface.
2. The operator should be in a position high enough above the patient that pressure can be exerted downward primarily by the weight of his body, rather than by arm motion. The most common mistake in administration of external cardiac massage is that the operator is too low and most of the force used in moving the patient's chest (and, secondarily, the heart) is exerted primarily by the operator's arms. There are very few persons who can maintain physical motion of the arms well enough to provide adequate thrust upon the chest.
3. Pressure should be exerted only over the lower one-third of the sternum, and contact with the sternum should be made with the heel of the hand

and *not* with the fingers. In most patients who do not have a calcified or fixed chest wall, satisfactory cardiac output can be maintained by depressing the sternum one to two inches.

4. Palpation of a pulse, usually a carotid or femoral pulse, will provide a rough estimate as to the effectiveness of cardiac massage. If the ventilation and cardiac perfusion by external cardiac massage are adequate, the pupillary response to light should be restored.

5. The heart should be compressed at a rate of 60 times per minute, giving a ratio of ventilation to perfusion of 1 : 4. A good team effort by two persons can adequately accomplish this vital task.

6. External cardiac massage with ventilation should be continuous except for *momentary* interruptions to obtain an electrocardiogram or to defibrillate the patient's heart. They should be stopped only when spontaneous, effective cardiac output has been restored or when a decision has been made by a physician to abandon the resuscitation.

Although seemingly complicated, the management of severe allergic reactions should be a matter of routine for anyone administering contrast materials. The first few seconds may be the most important time of that patient's life.

READING LIST

General

Physicians' Desk Reference for Radiology and Nuclear Medicine. Oradell, N. J.: Medical Economics, Inc., 1971.
Radiopaque Media. In *American Medical Association Drug Evaluation.* Chicago: American Medical Association, 1971.
Strain, W. H. (Ed.). Radiologic Diagnostic Agents. *Med. Radiogr. Photogr.* (Suppl.) 40, 1964.

Specific

Bernstein, E. R., and Gans, H. Anticoagulant activity of angiographic contrast media. *Invest. Radiol.* 1:162, 1966.
Fischer, H. W. Angiographic contrast mediums. *Postgrad. Med.* 43:59, 1968.
Fischer, H. W. Hemodynamic reaction to angiographic media. *Radiology* 91:66, 1968.
Fischer, H. W., and Cornell, S. H. The toxicity of sodium and methylglucamine salts of diatrizoate, iothalamate, and metrizoate. *Radiology* 85:1013, 1965.
Lasser, E. C. Basic mechanisms of contrast media reactions. *Radiology* 91:63, 1968.
Lillehei, C. W., Lavadia, P. G., DeWall, R. A., and Sellers, R. D. Four years' experience with external cardiac resuscitation. *J.A.M.A.* 193:651, 1965.
National Research Council. Cardiopulmonary resuscitation. *J.A.M.A.* 198:138, 1966.
Ross, R. J., and Bodie, J. F. A clinical evaluation of drip infusion urography. *Ohio State Med. J.* 64:1359, 1968.
Sanger, M. D. Further observations with antihistamines in reducing reactions in intravenous pyelography. *Ann. Allergy* 17:762, 1959.

Scheneker, B. Drip infusion pyelography. *Radiology* 83:12, 1964.
Sisel, R. J., Donovan, A. J., and Yellin, A. E. Experimental fecal peritonitis. *Arch. Surg.*
        104:765, 1972.

Basic Elements of Topographical Anatomy and X-ray Positioning

4

IT IS STANDARD in most radiology departments to take at least two different views of each area of interest. Because of superimposition, magnification, and distortion found in some views, pathological changes may be hidden on one view but readily seen on others. Demonstrations of the value of multiple views will be appreciated in forthcoming sections. One must imagine anatomy in three dimensions to be able to apply the radiological concepts presented here and to understand the fundamentals of diagnostic radiology.

Knowledge of basic x-ray positioning and topographical anatomy is essential in order that the student can communicate with other members of the health-care team. Certain landmarks noted on the human body are used to identify regions of interest. The terminology is standard, used by all members of the health-care team, and should be committed to memory.

It is important that the physician, paramedic, or any person requesting roentgenograms (also called radiographs) communicate with the radiological technologist as exactly as possible what the clinician is looking for. It is frustrating for radiological technologists to attempt a skull series on an agitated patient or to try to obtain a prone abdominal film on a patient with recent abdominal surgery.

By appreciating the basic elements of topographical anatomy and x-ray positioning, the student will be able to provide better medical service to the patient.

TOPOGRAPHICAL ANATOMY

The human body is divided by three common anatomical planes describing areas of interest (Fig. 4-1). An imaginary plane dividing the body into right and left

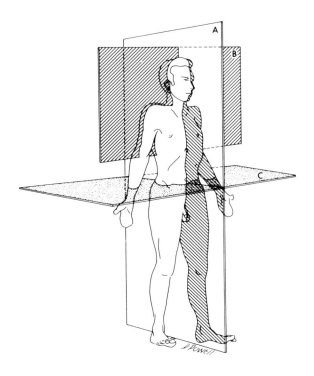

Fig. 4-1.
Anatomical planes. A, sagittal; B, coronal; C, transverse.

halves is termed the *sagittal plane.* Separation of the body into anterior and
posterior parts by another imaginary plane is termed the *frontal* or *coronal plane.*
A transverse plane divides the body into superior and inferior aspects.

As a matter of convenience, the body is divided into head, neck, trunk, and
upper and lower extremities. The head includes the skull and facial soft tissues.
The neck encloses the cervical vertebrae, connecting the head to the trunk. The
trunk includes the thorax, abdomen, and pelvis. The upper extremities consist
of the shoulders, arms, forearms, and hands. The lower extremities consist of
the hips, thighs, legs, and feet. Each of these primary topographical regions has
a number of subdivisions.

The topographical regions of the head correspond to the underlying bony
structures (Fig. 4-2). The cranial portion of the skull encases the brain and is
subdivided into the frontal (anterior), parietal (posterosuperior), occipital (posterior), and temporal (lateral) areas. The temporal areas also include the auricular
appendages and mastoid regions.

The facial structures include the regions of the eyes (orbital), nose (nasal),
mouth (oral), cheeks (buccal), and jaws (mandibular, middle). The upper jaws

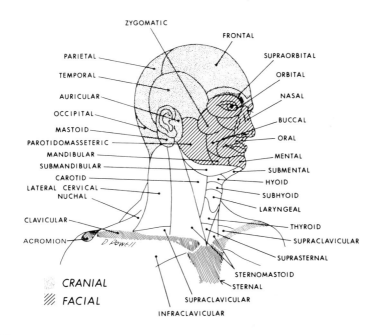

Fig. 4-2.
Topographical regions of the head and neck.

contribute to portions of other facial structures and are not considered separate
entities. The paranasal sinuses underlie the facial structures.

As with the cranium, the neck has superficial regions named for their relationship to adjacent structures. The *nuchal area* indicates the back of the neck and
overlies the posterior spinous processes of the cervical vertebrae. The side portion
of the neck is referred to as the *lateral cervical area;* anteriorly, one refers to the
anterior cervical region. The clavicles demarcate the inferior portion of the neck,
and this region is referred to as the *clavicular area.* Immediately superior to this
area is the supraclavicular area, which is lateral to the sternocleidomastoid muscle.
The small infraclavicular areas are just inferior to the clavicles. Each of these
regions is subdivided as noted in Figure 4-2.

The trunk is composed of the thorax, abdomen, and pelvis (Fig. 4-3). The
thorax consists of a wall enclosing the thoracic cavity and its contents. The
skeletal components of the wall include the sternum, twelve pairs of ribs, and
twelve thoracic vertebrae. The thoracic viscera include the heart, lungs, and
great vessels. Externally, the anterior chest is divided into right and left pectoral regions separated by the sternum. The mammary glands (breasts) are super-
ficially located in the lower pectoral regions. Just superior to the pectoral
regions are the small infraclavicular regions. On the posterior thorax the main

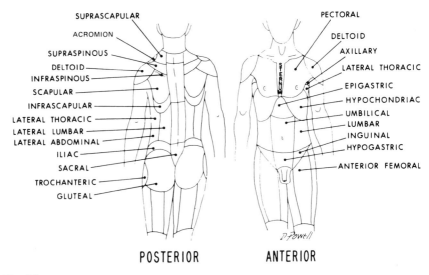

Fig. 4-3.
Topographical regions of the trunk.

areas of interest include the regions of the scapulae and the infrascapular
areas.

The abdomen is that part of the trunk which lies between the thorax and
the pelvis. The abdomen encloses the gastrointestinal tract, liver, spleen, pancreas, kidneys, and adrenal glands. The thoracic and abdominal cavities are
separated anatomically and perhaps functionally by the diaphragm. Because of
the dome-shaped configuration of the diaphragm, some of the abdominal viscera,
particularly the spleen and liver, may actually lie within the thoracic portion of
the trunk, since these organs may on occasion extend above the level of the rib
margins. Hence, there is an overlap between the lower thoracic viscera, the lungs,
and the upper abdominal viscera, the spleen and liver.

The anterior abdominal wall is divided into nine topographical regions as
noted in Figure 4-3. The epigastric region is that area just below the sternum
and overlying the stomach. The two hypochondriac regions are essentially the
lower portions of the rib cage. In the midabdominal area the quadrant about
the umbilicus is termed the *umbilical region,* with the two lateral regions termed
the *lumbar regions.* Inferiorly, the two inguinal regions overlie the inguinal
ligaments, with the midportion overlying the bladder termed the *hypogastric
region.* These regions are extremely important in describing locations of pain
and possible mass lesions.

There is also a sharing of the pelvic and abdominal cavities by crucial organs,
with a portion of the bowel being noted in the pelvis and a portion of the female

reproductive glands being located in the abdomen. The pelvis is divided into an upper part, called the *false pelvis,* and a lower portion, the *true pelvis.* In actual practice the major pelvis is generally treated as part of the abdominal cavity. Other important organs located in the pelvis include the urinary bladder, uterus, and sigmoid colon.

Several imaginary lines are noted on the anterior trunk. The midsternal line is an imaginary line drawn from the sternal notch through the umbilicus to the symphysis pubis. Paralleling these lines are the lateral sternal lines, which are located at the lateral borders of the sternum. The midclavicular line begins at the midportion of the clavicle and extends down toward the pelvis.

At the site of attachment to the trunk, both superior and inferior extremities have some transition between the regions of the trunk and the extremities. Thus, the axilla has part of its surface on the lateral wall of the thorax and part on the medial surface of the arm in the region of the brachium. The scapular region, also classified as part of the back, is related to the arm because it also includes the muscles with their humeral attachments. Similarly, the buttocks adjacent to the bones of the pelvis contain muscles which act upon the lower limbs.

The topographical anatomy of the upper extremities is noted in Figure 4-4. Of particular interest is the antecubital fossa, which is the anterior portion of the elbow and the soft tissues of the palm of the hand overlying the thumb and fifth metacarpal, termed *thenar* and *hypothenar* areas, respectively. One should also note that *palmar* refers to the palm of the hand and *dorsum* refers to the back

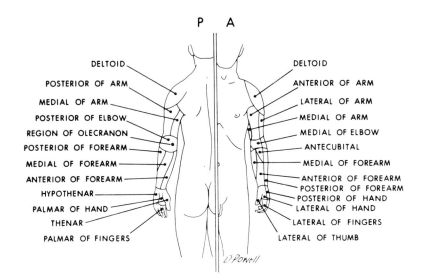

Fig. 4-4.

Topographical regions of the upper limb, or extremity.

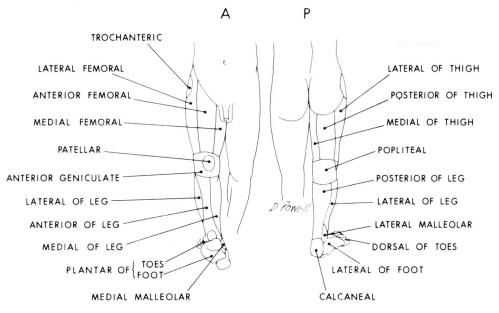

Fig. 4-5.
Topographical regions of the lower limb, or extremity.

of the hand. In actual practice, one refers to the region of the distal forearm as the *wrist.* Figure 4-5 depicts the topographical anatomy of the lower extremity. Again, *dorsum* refers to the top of the foot and *plantar* refers to the sole of the foot and toes.

The perineal region includes the anal, urogenital, and pudendal areas. Figure 4-6 depicts these areas.

FUNDAMENTAL X-RAY POSITIONING

The old Chinese proverb which states that "a picture is worth a thousand words" has particular significance in radiology. In teaching basic radiology to allied health personnel and medical students, one becomes painfully aware that many students have no concept of how certain basic roentgenograms are produced in the radiology department. Only by clearly understanding the basic positions in which patients are placed to be x-rayed can one project what should be anticipated from a particular study. Volumes have been written concerning the positioning of patients for roentgenograms, but only a few basic positions need to be understood for one to appreciate the majority of everyday roentgenographic procedures. In addition, certain terms applicable not only to the

PERINEAL REGION

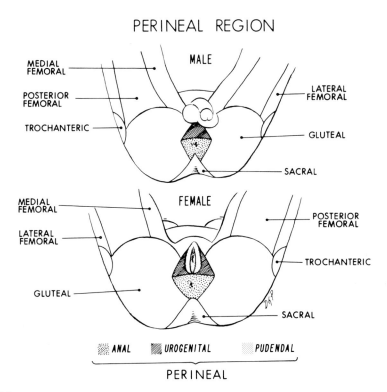

Fig. 4-6.
Topographical areas of the perineal region.

specialty of radiology but to others, as well, enhance one's ability to interpret roentgenographic reports and to request roentgenographic examinations in an intelligent manner. Only by understanding words or terms peculiar to a field of interest can one effectively communicate with others in that field.

The following x-ray positions indicate how the roentgenogram is made, how the resultant film may be imaginarily superimposed on the patient's body, and how one views that film, so that the student can appreciate that particular projection. By convention, certain letters are commonly used which the reader should commit to memory. *P* stands for "posterior" and indicates that the x-ray beam enters or exits through the posterior portion of the area being examined. *A* is the reverse in that the x-ray beam enters or exits anteriorly. For example, *PA* implies a posterior x-ray beam which exits anteriorly. *R* is for "right," and *L* is for "left." *O* applies to "oblique." *Upright* implies that the patient was in the upright position when the roentgenogram was exposed. *Prone* indicates that the patient was lying on his stomach; *supine,* lying on his back.

Decubitus indicates lying on the side. Other basic projections will be indicated as that area of the body is studied.

Chest Films. The standard position for half the chest roentgenograms made in the United States is PA, or posteroanterior (Fig. 4-7). This roentgenogram is made with a six-foot focal—film distance and a horizontal x-ray beam. The patient's chest is placed against a film cassette with the x-ray beam striking the

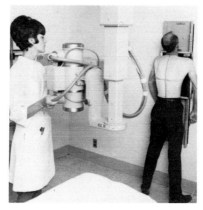

Normal x-ray position

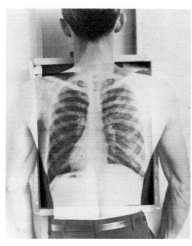

Normal exposed film

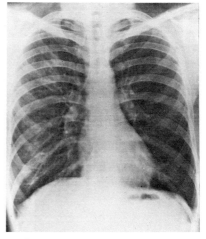

Proper viewing of completed film

Fig. 4-7.
   Posteroanterior chest film.

back and exiting anteriorly. The vast majority of these films are made with the patient in the upright position, although on rare occasions the film may be made with the patient lying on a stretcher or table. The reason for taking a routine PA chest film rather than an AP film is that the heart is anteriorly situated in the thorax and less magnification of the heart thus results.

The lateral chest film (Fig. 4-8) is generally exposed with the left side of the chest against the film cassette. Since the heart is slightly to the left of the midline, there is slightly less magnification of the heart when a left lateral is obtained as opposed to a right lateral film.

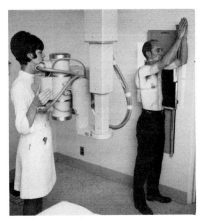

Normal x-ray position

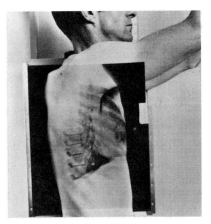

Normal exposed film

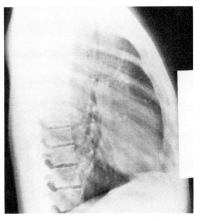

Proper viewing of completed film

Fig. 4-8.
Left lateral chest film.

The lateral chest film is used to examine the thoracic spine and cardiac size and particularly to localize lesions which may have been seen on the PA chest film. It is difficult for most radiological technologists to obtain a true lateral chest film, but rotation of the patient becomes important in evaluating cardiac chamber size. Obliquity can be appreciated by noting the superimposition of the posterior ribs on one another.

The AP chest film is obtained when it is impractical to obtain a PA film. Although one occasionally obtains a standing AP film, it is more common for the patient to be sitting, as in a wheelchair, or lying in bed when this view is obtained. Anteroposterior films may be obtained with the patient lying on the x-ray table or by the use of a portable x-ray machine. X-ray equipment in general use prohibits a six-foot overhead focal—film distance, and the standard distance for an AP chest film is 36 to 42 inches. Obviously from the introduction to basic x-ray physics in Chapter 2 one would infer there is more magnification on an AP chest film projected by tabletop or portable x-ray equipment.

Decubitus films may also be obtained of the chest. This projection is to demonstrate free fluid or air in the thorax or to detect movement of mass lesions. If fluid is suspected in the right pleural space, a right lateral decubitus film should be obtained, and vice versa. However, if air—fluid levels are to be demonstrated, it is usually wise to obtain the opposite decubitus view, as there would be less film fog and distortion of that portion of the body away from the x-ray tabletop. Suspected pathology determines the position in which the roentgenogram is exposed.

Portable chest films leave much to be desired as far as quality is concerned. These films are generally obtained only on the most seriously ill patients who cannot control their respiratory effort to any degree, and the equipment used to obtain the roentgenograms is mostly of small capacity which cannot produce the short exposure times needed to stop motion from being recorded on the film. The end result from most portable roentgenograms is a poor film with limited detail taken of a critically ill patient for whose case the radiologist should have had the best diagnostic film possible.

Apical lordotic films (Fig. 4-9) are obtained either by having the patient stand about a foot in front of the film cassette and lean backward against the film cassette or by having the patient stand erect, with the x-ray beam tilted. A tilted or horizontal beam is used at a six-foot focal—film distance. This examination is used to evaluate the apexes of the lung, the right middle lobe, and the lingula of the left upper lobe. In this position, the clavicles are projected superiorly to the apexes of the lungs and the anterior ribs are superimposed on the posterior ribs.

The right anterior oblique (RAO, Fig. 4-10) and the left anterior oblique (LAO, Fig. 4-11) projections are PA films of different obliquity which are used primarily for cardiac evaluation and examination of the esophagus. Obliques may also be used to localize lesions within the chest, but unfortu-

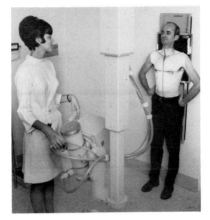

Normal x-ray position

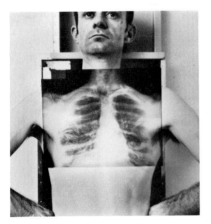

Normal exposed film

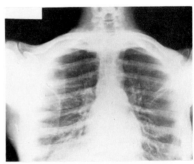

Proper viewing of completed film

Fig. 4-9.
Apical lordotic chest film. This film may also be obtained by using a horizontal x-ray beam and having the patient lean backward against the film cassette.

nately they are not commonly used by radiologists. The LAO for cardiac evaluation is of 60 degrees' rotation, made with the left shoulder against the film cassette; and the RAO is of 45 degrees' obliquity, with the right shoulder against the cassette. Again, it is important to obtain the proper rotations to evaluate cardiac size. The LAO is also particularly useful in examining the course of the thoracic aorta. Both projections are used in examining the barium-filled esophagus for displacement and intrinsic or extrinsic filling defects.

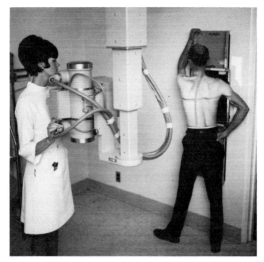

Normal x-ray position

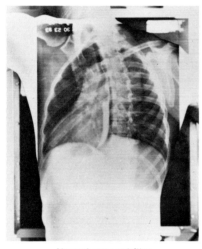

Normal exposed film

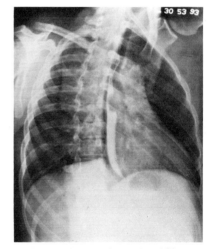

Proper viewing of completed film

Fig. 4-10.

Right anterior oblique chest film. Note the barium-filled esophagus.

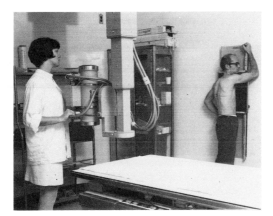

Normal x-ray position

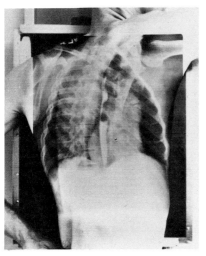

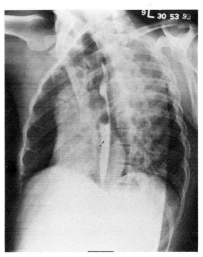

Normal exposed film   Proper viewing of completed film

Fig. 4-11.
Left anterior oblique chest film. In examining the cardiac silhouette, the esophagus is not filled with barium since it may obscure detail in the region of the left atrial appendage.

Abdominal Films. Figures 4-12 and 4-13 illustrate the common examinations used for evaluation of the abdomen, namely the obstructive series. The flat plate of the abdomen is made with the patient supine and the x-ray beam centered in midabdomen. The intestinal gas pattern, renal and psoas shadows, bony struc-tures, presence of calculi and hepatic and splenic size are thus demonstrated. The patient is then tilted up on the x-ray table and a film is exposed to demonstrate

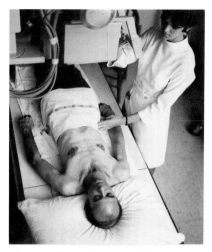

Normal x-ray position

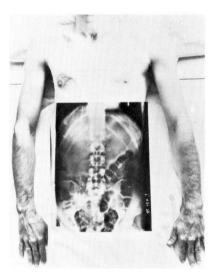

Normal exposed film

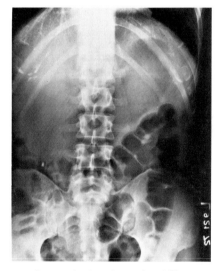

Proper viewing of completed film

Fig. 4-12.
*K*idney, *u*reter, and *b*ladder (KUB) or flat plate or AP view of the abdomen. Note the gas in the stomach. Air—fluid levels may be used to indicate in which position the x-ray film was exposed.

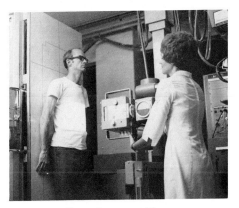

Normal x-ray position

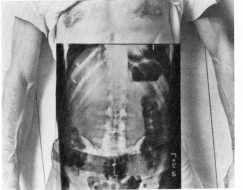

Normal exposed film

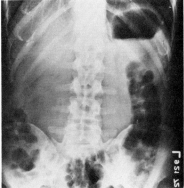

Proper viewing of completed film

Fig. 4-13.
   Upright abdominal film. Note the air—fluid level in the stomach. On the normal exposed film, the belt and clothing were purposely left on to demonstrate why clothing should be removed before x-raying an area.

the presence of air—fluid levels within loops of bowel. If the patient is too ill to tolerate being in the upright position, however, a lateral decubitus film (Fig. 4-14) of the abdomen may be obtained with a horizontal x-ray beam. One must be aware that the patient should be in the lateral decubitus or upright position for approximately 5 to 10 minutes before the film is exposed in order to allow free air in the peritoneal cavity to gravitate to its free position. Occasionally, a cross-table lateral roentgenogram of the abdomen may be obtained which shows the same general information as the lateral decubitus or upright abdominal film. This is used mainly to localize abdominal masses.

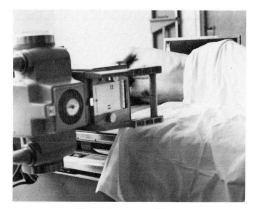

Normal x-ray position

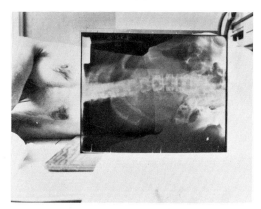

Normal exposed film

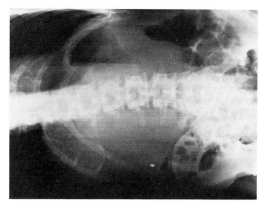

Proper viewing of completed film

Fig. 4-14.
Right lateral decubitus film. Again, note the air—fluid level in the stomach.

48

Skull Films. A skull series consists of a variable number of projections chosen to demonstrate a particular area of interest or as a survey of the cranium. Many of the projections, especially those of the temporal bone, are very difficult to interpret and seemingly complicated for radiological technologists to position and expose properly. A select series is presented, and the anatomy will be discussed later.

In positioning the skull for roentgenograms, a constant landmark should be understood. This topographical landmark is termed the *orbital-meatal line* and is an imaginary line drawn from the outer canthus of the eye to the center of the external auditory meatus. Reference will be made to this landmark in the discussion of the positions in which the head is placed before exposing films of the skull. The student should appreciate from the illustrations how difficult it would be to obtain an appropriate set of skull films on an agitated patient, as well as the danger of requesting a complete skull series in patients with suspected cervical fractures.

The PA skull film (Fig. 4-15) is exposed with the x-ray beam parallel to the orbital-meatal line and exiting at the base of the nose. This projection allows good visualization of the ethmoidal sinuses, orbits, petrous ridges and tips, cranial vault, and pineal gland.

The Towne view (Fig. 4-16) is made with an AP x-ray beam angulated 23 to 35 degrees caudally to the orbital-meatal line. This angulation casts the facial bones downward, exposing the posterior fossa and the temporal bones for examination. The sella is generally well seen, and the temporal bones are elongated, affording good visualization.

The lateral film (Fig. 4-17) is made with the right or left side of the cranium against the film cassette and with the x-ray beam centered at the external ear canal and exiting at the same level on the opposite side. This view allows one to examine the cranial vault in toto — the anterior, middle, and posterior fossae; the sella; the pineal gland; and the facial bones.

The base plate, or submental vertex (Fig. 4-18) is exposed with the x-ray beam perpendicular to the orbital-meatal line. It is used for evaluation of the foramina, sinuses, orbits, and temporal bone anatomy.

The Water's view (Fig. 4-19) is used to examine the facial bones primarily, including the paranasal sinuses. It is made with a PA x-ray beam with the chin placed against the film cassette and the nose slightly elevated from the surface of the cassette. A stereoscopic Water's view is the most appropriate film to request for evaluation of facial trauma.

Although most radiologists prefer to obtain skull films with a neuroradiological head unit such as the Franklin head unit demonstrated in the illustrations, the same projections can be obtained from tabletop positioning. However, it should be noted that the films of the paranasal sinuses should be obtained in the upright position in order to demonstrate air—fluid levels and that at least one lateral view of the skull should be obtained with a cross-table

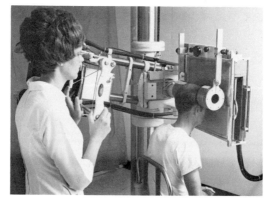

Normal x-ray position

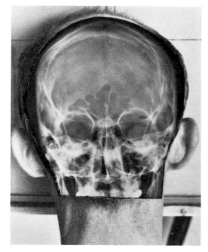

Normal exposed film   Proper viewing of completed film

Fig. 4-15.
Posteroanterior skull projection. In many radiology departments the x-ray beam may be tilted 12 to 15 degrees caudally to delineate the middle fossa structures better.

beam when trauma is suspected in order to demonstrate air—fluid levels in the sphenoidal sinuses.

Pelvic Films. The remaining common x-ray position is the flat plate of the pelvis (Fig. 4-20). This film is made with the patient supine, although on occasion the film is made PA. The x-ray beam is centered at the level of the symphysis pubis, and a 14- by 17-inch film is exposed. This allows visualization

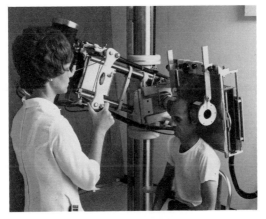

Normal x-ray position

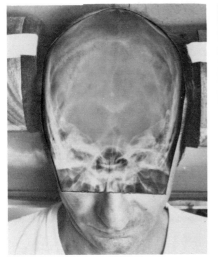

Normal exposed film

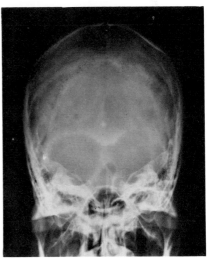

Proper viewing of completed film

Fig. 4-16.
  Anteroposterior Towne view. Notice the tilt of the x-ray beam.

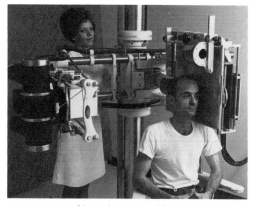

Normal x-ray position

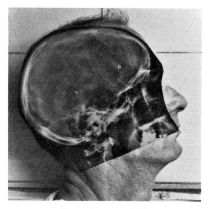 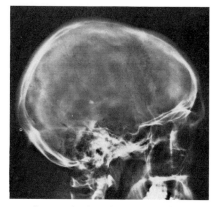

Normal exposed film   Proper viewing of completed film

Fig. 4-17.
Lateral skull film.

of the lower lumbar spine, sacroiliac joints, hips, and soft tissues of the pelvis. In examining the hips at a different angle from that projected on the AP film, the legs are drawn upward and the heels are placed together. This position is termed a *frog-leg lateral* (Fig. 4-21), and the position of the legs as demonstrated in the illustration forces abduction of the hips, providing a right-angle view of the femoral heads. This is particularly useful in examining children.

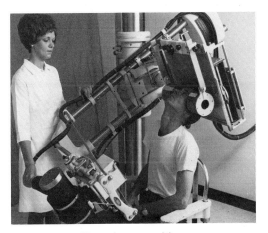

Normal x-ray position

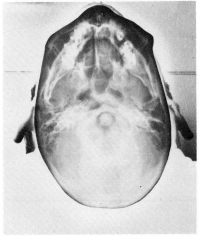

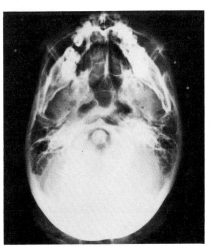

Normal exposed film   Proper viewing of completed film

Fig. 4-18.

Submental vertex film. By varying the tilt of the x-ray beam, different areas of the base of the skull may be visualized better than others.

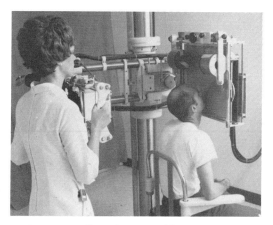

Normal x-ray position

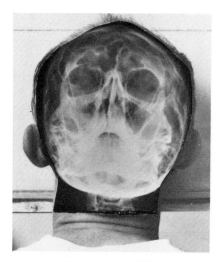

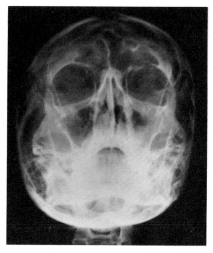

Normal exposed film   Proper viewing of completed film

Fig. 4-19.
Water's view of the skull. The facial bones are well demonstrated, but a stereoscopic view will allow one to recognize fractures that may not be so apparent on a single film.

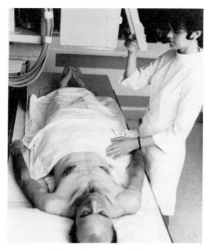

Normal x-ray position

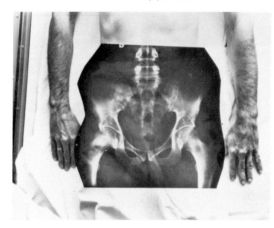

Normal exposed film

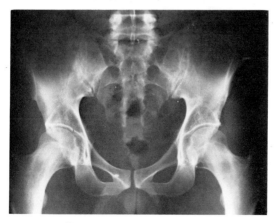

Proper viewing of completed film

Fig. 4-20.
Anteroposterior film of the pelvis.

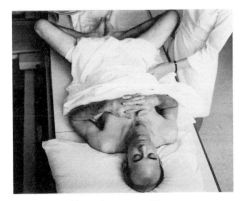

Normal x-ray position

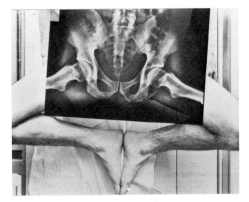

Normal exposed film

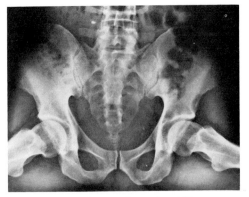

Proper viewing of completed film

Fig. 4-21.
Frog-leg lateral film of the pelvis.

The Osseous System

5

UP TO THIS POINT there has deliberately been no mention of techniques for examining roentgenograms. In examining the osseous system, there is a marked contrast between the densities of bones and soft tissues, so that the student has little difficulty in discerning different shades of gray demarcating the adjacent structures. It would be well to establish some rules for the student to follow when examining roentgenograms.

PRINCIPLES IN EXAMINING ROENTGENOGRAMS

The art of communication dictates that one convey a distinct thought to another with minimal loss of detail. Innate ability, intellectual ability, and experience combine to allow some to communicate better than others. The communication of graphic detail to a referring physician is the role of the radiologist. In describing roentgenographic detail, the radiologist must avoid vocabulary which is not in general usage and be as direct and succinct as possible in relaying his impressions to the referring physician.

Although allied health workers should not be relied upon to make diagnoses from roentgenograms, they should be capable of scanning most routine films and picking up gross abnormalities for the physician employer in order to expedite patient care. Interpretation of roentgenographic studies is the responsibility of radiologists and should not be delegated to other persons, be they physicians or nonphysicians.

A roentgenogram provides an infinite number of facts. It has been said, for example, that a single PA chest film contains over one hundred million bits of information. The assimilation of these facts allows one to arrive at an impression. Correlation of the roentgenographic impression with medical histories and physical examination data allows one to arrive at a diagnosis. It is, therefore, rather obvious that one should be able to arrive at an impression from any roentgeno-graphic study; but to arrive at a diagnosis may be next to impossible. The more experience and training one has, the more facts he can obtain from a roentgeno-graphic study and hence the more accurate his impression or diagnosis will be. It should be noted that the ability of a radiologist to obtain facts from a roent-genographic study varies from time to time and ultimately will lead to different impressions or diagnoses from the same study on different occasions.

In examining roentgenograms, there can be no substitute for developing a system for complete study of the film. This technique may vary from one par-ticular study to another, but one must adhere to a few basic premises no matter what examination is being reviewed.

1. Make absolutely certain that the roentgenogram in question is actually that of the patient being evaluated. If the film is not marked with the patient's name, ascribed number, or other identifying marks, never accept it as belonging to that particular patient. It is less expensive to repeat the film than to pay legal costs for a malpractice suit. Patients do not appre-ciate being treated for something they do not have.
2. Make sure right is right and left is left. The heart is not always on the left side, and the liver is not always on the right. One still hears of fractures being treated on the wrong side of the body.
3. Do not limit the examination to the area of interest. Films contain four corners, and all four should be examined. It is rather embarrassing to re-port a chest film as normal when a dislocated humeral head is also present.
4. Two views of every part examined are mandatory. Too often a carcinoma of the lung can be seen on a lateral view but not on the PA view. Fractures may be seen on one view and not on another.
5. Particularly in examination of extremities for trauma, the joint above and the joint below the area of trauma must be x-rayed. Cursory examination of a patient complaining of trauma to the ankle may cause one to overlook a fractured fibular head.
6. Roentgenograms must be of the utmost quality, properly centered, and adequately collimated for radiation protection. This presupposes that the examination is performed by a well-trained, qualified radiologist or radio-logic technologist.

Following the above cardinal rules will usually prevent one from making a major mistake. Adherence to these basic principles is mandatory for good radiology.

Since radiology is generally the application of medical knowledge to gross anatomy, prerequisites are a good general working knowledge of anatomy and physiology and a basic understanding of medical maladies. A meager knowledge of either cannot be supplanted by a greater knowledge of the other prerequisite.

As a corollary to previewing roentgenograms, the necessity of obtaining roentgenographic studies in the proper sequence must be reemphasized. To request an excretory urogram before radionuclide studies on a patient suspected of hyperthyroidism is inexcusable. Radionuclide examination of the thyroid gland should be performed before administration of any water-soluble contrast material: hence barium enema studies are done before upper gastrointestinal studies, urograms before barium studies, films of the lumbosacral spine before barium studies, and so on. Haphazard requests for radiographic studies cannot substitute for a carefully planned diagnostic regimen.

BONY TRAUMA

The allied health worker will be concerned with trauma to the osseous system more than to any other pathological entity. Hence, most of our discussion of the osseous system will relate to fractures. A brief discussion of some of the more common diseases of bone will also be included for completeness.

It is presumed that the student in radiology has an adequate background knowledge of what causes a fracture, what a fracture is, and how it heals. To summarize, when a fracture occurs there is a break in the endosteum and periosteum and some degree of damage to nearby soft tissues. Surrounding vessels are disrupted, and the adjacent tissues are infiltrated with blood, lymph, and tissue fluid. Swelling results, causing pain which is increased by movement at the fracture site. There also may be associated injury to nearby nerves, blood vessels, and viscera; and the physical examination must include these areas since the radiographic examination often will not show them. Fractures of large bones may lead to a greater blood loss than one would anticipate and can result in vascular shock. It is not uncommon for a liter of blood to be lost into the surrounding tissues following a fracture of the femoral shaft.

Fractures heal in a prescribed manner. Blood, lymph, and tissue fluid accumulate and surround the fracture site, forming a fibrin clot. Fibroblasts appear shortly and begin formation of granulation tissue, ultimately becoming organized tissue which stabilizes the fracture. Calcium is deposited in this new tissue, producing callus formation; and with use and normal stress, the bone rearranges its line and channels and may ultimately appear as normal. The length of time required for repair of bony trauma is affected by the age, health, and nutrition of the patient and by the circulation to the fracture site. Children heal rapidly, usually without deformity; whereas adults in poor health and with poor circulation may never adequately heal. Location and vascular supply may affect the healing; certain areas such as the subcapital and intracapsular areas of the femoral neck, the junction of the lower and middle thirds of the tibia, the proximal portion of the carpal navicular, and the lower third of the ulna are sites that have a particular tendency to heal poorly and that should have prolonged immobilization.

Certain definitions are also prerequisite to a general consideration of bony trauma. A fracture is *complete* when it involves the entire cross section of bone and *incomplete* if it does not. A *closed* fracture does not break the skin and is not exposed to outside air. *Transverse, spiral,* and *oblique* describe the direction of the line of fracture in relation to the long axis of the bone involved. A *comminuted* fracture has two or more lines which divide the fracture into three or more parts. An *impacted* fracture is present when one fragment is driven firmly into the other. *Pathological* fractures occur through an area of abnormal or diseased bone. *Dislocation* implies that the bone is "out of joint" and is no longer in contact with its normal articulation. *Subluxation* is a partial dislocation.

Fractures are also described as to the angulation of the distal fragment in relation to the proximal fragment, whether the alignment is satisfactory, and whether adequate bony apposition is present.

Complications of fractures may be insignificant or disabling. *Delayed union* implies that healing did not occur within the time usually allotted for a fracture of that particular type. *Malunion* signifies that healing occurred in such a manner as to impair normal function or cosmetic appearance. *Nonunion* occurs when the healing process stops without union of the fragments. Severance of major blood vessels or nerves, cosmetic deformity, avascular necrosis of bone, and contractures may all result from bony trauma.

The most frequent reason for roentgenographic examination of the extremities is to detect fractures. Most fractures are easily identifiable, but one must be constantly aware that a fracture may be noted on one film and not on another. The clinician usually notices fractures of the extremities readily, particularly when the cardinal signs of pain, swelling, deformity, and cramping are present. These signs are not seen in all fractures; and joint fractures commonly masquerade as sprains, or vice versa. It is in the best interests of the patient to x-ray all areas of suspected bone trauma.

For the sake of better communication, fractures are described by their roentgenographic appearance. A few words concerning this and illustrations of the basic types of fractures are included below, and the student is referred to the references for more detail.

Greenstick Fractures. These fractures occur mostly in children. During bony development, the cancellous bone is soft and prone to bend or crack. As in a green tree limb, the fracture appears as a break in the cortex of one side of the bony shaft without separation or break of the opposite cortex. The distal radius is quite prone to such fractures; and in this area the cortex folds back upon itself, producing a *torus* fracture (Fig. 5-1).

Fatigue Fractures. These fractures occur at sites of maximum stress on bone, most often in the midportion of the metatarsals and occasionally in the lower extremities and lower ribs. They occur without evidence of trauma. Roent-

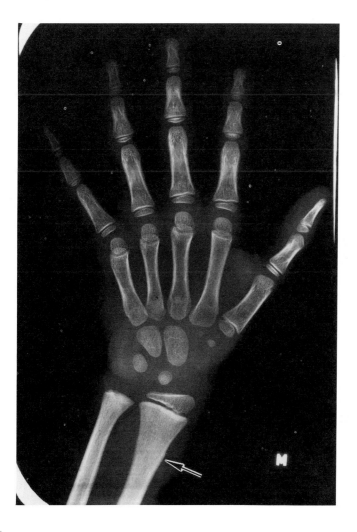

Fig. 5-1.
Greenstick fracture. Notice the slight irregularity of the cortex of the distal radius. On occasion, this may be the only sign of this type of fracture.

genographically, a hairline fracture may be noted; or on occasion, no fracture may be seen initially but subsequent films show bone resorption around the fracture followed by deposition of callus. These fractures are also known as *march* fractures, since they were commonly seen among soldiers after long, forced marches. They may also be seen in persons whose jobs require a great deal of walking; for example, nurses and postmen (Fig. 5-2).

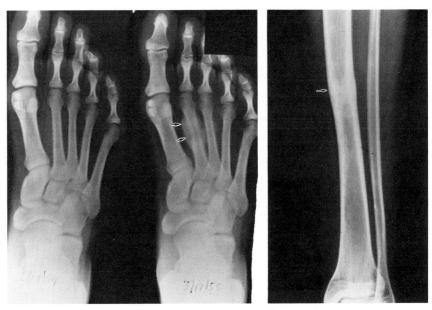

A   B

Fig. 5-2.

Fatigue fractures. (A) This was a 20-year-old college student who had come to the emergency room complaining of pain in his foot following a basketball game. No abnormality could be demonstrated on the roentgenogram. The pain continued; and the student was seen three months later, at which time the x-rays demonstrated a typical "fatigue" fracture.

(B) Occasionally the only roentgen sign of such a fracture is increased cortical thickness, as noted in this film taken some time after the fracture. The patient had given a history of persistent tibial pain for several months previously, but roentgenograms at the time were interpreted as being normal.

Pathological Fractures. Pathological fractures occur when normal stress is placed on abnormal bone (Fig. 5-3). When the stress exceeds the capability of the bone to withstand it, a fracture results. Many entities contribute to these fractures; and the exact cause of the fracture must be ascertained, since the underlying pathology must also be treated for successful healing to be achieved. Bone cysts, metastatic tumors, malacic metabolic bone diseases, primary bone tumors, osteomyelitis, and congenital bony defects are commonly associated with pathological fractures.

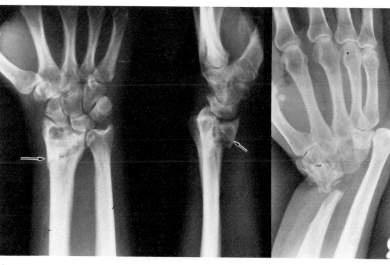

A

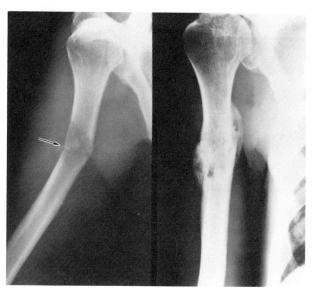

B

Fig. 5-3.
   Pathological fractures. (A) Fracture through a malignant giant cell tumor of the wrist. The tumor was resected, and the film on the right was made some fifteen years later.
   (B) Fracture through a metastatic renal tumor. The film on the right shows callus formation in response to the fracture.

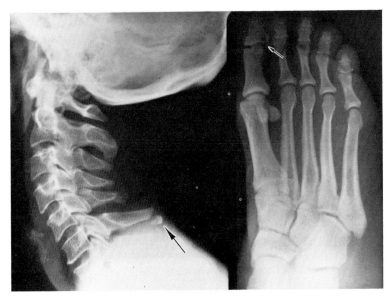

Fig. 5-4.
Typical chip fractures. The cervical fracture was secondary to an automobile accident.
The chip fracture of the distal phalanx of the toe resulted from a film cassette being dropped
on it.

Avulsion or Chip Fractures. These small fractures usually occur about joints
and are commonly associated with concomitant tearing of ligaments or tendons
or both (Fig. 5-4). They are also commonly seen in association with dislocations.

Epiphyseal Fractures. As the name implies, these fractures occur through an
unfused or un-united epiphysis and usually involve a small portion of the
metaphysis. Since many of these fractures occur without displacement, suspect
areas should have companion views made of the opposite side for comparison.
Comparison views of this type of fracture are considered mandatory (Fig. 5-5).

Spiral Fractures. Oblique or spiral fractures result from a rotary-type injury
to a long bone (Fig. 5-6). Frequently these fractures may be accompanied by
fractures elsewhere; and one must be certain to x-ray all suspect areas. If
necessary, additional films should also be obtained.

Impacted (T or Y) Fractures. These fractures are associated with joint spaces
and occur as a result of force being transmitted through the long bones from
impactions. They are commonly seen in parachute jumpers and result from
falls in which the patient landed with full force on straightened legs or arms.

Compression Fractures. These fractures most often occur in the spine. They
may be secondary to metastatic tumor but more often are associated with
trauma or malacic bone diseases such as osteoporosis or multiple myeloma
(Fig. 5-7).

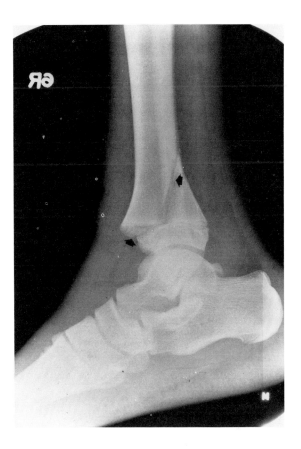

Fig. 5-5.
Epiphyseal fracture. There is an oblique fracture of the distal tibia (upper arrow).
An obvious epiphyseal fracture is also noted (lower arrow). Since bone growth occurs
through the epiphysis, epiphyseal fractures have the potential of being deforming.

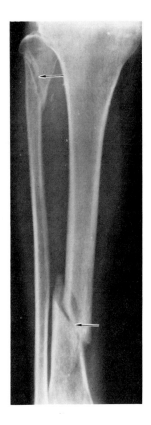

Fig. 5-6.

A partially healed oblique fracture through the proximal fibula and a recent spiral fracture through the distal tibia. Slight callus formation is seen surrounding the fibular fracture, and none is seen about the tibial fracture. The amount of callus formation present allows one to estimate how long ago the fracture occurred.

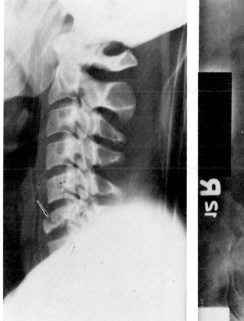

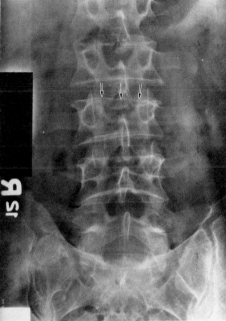

A

B

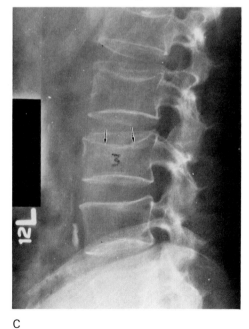

C

Fig. 5-7.

Compression fractures. (A) Compression fracture of C-6 following an automobile accident. (B) Compression fracture of L-3. (C) Lateral roentgenogram of the same patient as in (B). If one is careless, the fracture can easily be overlooked, as this one was.

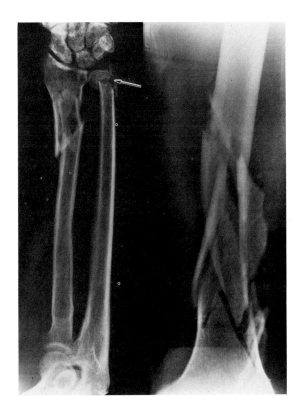

Fig. 5-8.
Comminuted fracture of the distal radius and of ulna and femur in different patients.

Comminuted Fractures. *Comminuted* means "crushed or broken into pieces." Severe trauma may result in comminuted fractures, and a bullet wound may also create severe destruction of the bone, which is called a *comminuted fracture* (Fig. 5-8).

Combined Fracture and Dislocation. The most common dislocations involve the shoulder, hip, and elbow. Other dislocations are almost invariably associated with fractures.

Shoulder dislocations are more common anteriorly and can be easily recognized roentgenographically (Fig. 5-9). These dislocations may be uncomplicated or may be associated with a chip fracture of the lower lip of the glenoid fossa and possible injury to nerves and vascular supply. Particular awareness of

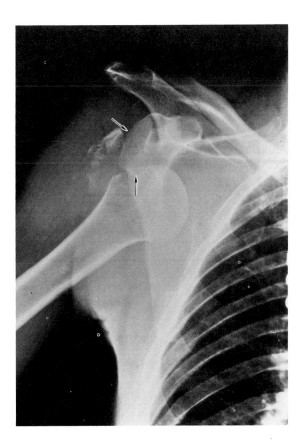

Fig. 5-9.
Anterior fracture and dislocation of the shoulder. The glenoid fossa is outlined by arrows.

possible injury to the nerves or vessels is mandatory when the reduction of these injuries is being performed.

Posterior dislocation is uncommon and may not be recognized either clinically or roentgenographically. Anterior dislocations locate the humeral head in the subglenoid fossa, which is easily recognized on the roentgenogram. However, the posterior dislocation may demonstrate the humeral head at the same level as the glenoid fossa; and one must obtain transaxillary films to demonstrate the exact location of the humeral head. If one suspects that a patient has a posterior dislocation, the transaxillary view should be requested since the PA film will not demonstrate this dislocation.

Dislocation of the hip may be simple, with the femoral head located posteriorly and lying against the sciatic notch. Occasionally an anterior displacement may show the femoral head adjacent to the pubic or obturator foramen. Intrapubic dislocation is always associated with a fracture of the acetabulum.

Congenital dislocation of the hip is most likely to be noted in the newborn nursery. Dislocations of this type are generally secondary to acetabular dysplasia or subluxation or both. Although usually used interchangeably for dislocation, *subluxation* means partially dislocated. Congenital dislocation is usually unilateral and is recognized by obvious shortening of one extremity. The piston sign, demonstrated by flexing the knee and forcibly alternating pushing and pulling the femur, is used in evaluating a congenital dislocation. If the hip is dislocated, the femoral head can be palpated through the gluteal muscles as it slides in and out of the acetabular cup. The dysplastic hip may not always appear as a shortened extremity, however; it may be suggested only by asymmetry of the gluteal folds, with occasional limited abduction of the hip.

Pediatric hip problems must be recognized and treated early. If the displaced hip is not recognized until the child begins to walk, conservative therapy is difficult; and beyond the age of 4 or 5, it almost certainly requires surgical intervention.

Acromioclavicular displacement or separation is more commonly seen in children. This occurs as a result of force applied to the outer shoulder. An obvious soft tissue bulge may be recognized in the acromioclavicular area. Roentgenographically, acromioclavicular separation can be demonstrated by having the patient stand while holding weights in each hand; and companion views of both shoulders will show the separation (Fig. 5-10). Widening of the acromioclavicular joint greater than 1 cm must be viewed with suspicion.

The foregoing is only a brief summary of the roentgenographic aspects of bony trauma. One should be aware of the medicolegal aspects of injuries; and it is safe to state that if there is any suggestion of bony trauma, radiographs should be obtained. Although on occasion fractures may be reduced without the need for roentgenographic analysis, it is in the best interests of the patient to obtain films before and after the reduction. No reduction should ever be attempted with only a single-view film.

NONNEOPLASTIC BONE CHANGES

Nonneoplastic bone disease includes a whole gamut of disease entities — the arthritides, osteitis, congenital dysplasias, and other metabolic or inherited bone abnormalities. Fortunately, in everyday practice only a few of these entities are seen; and the reader is referred to the Reading List for specific information regarding a particular entity.

Osteoporosis. Osteoporosis is an abnormal decrease in bone density due to failure of osteoblasts to lay down bone matrix. Clinically, *osteoporosis* is sometimes

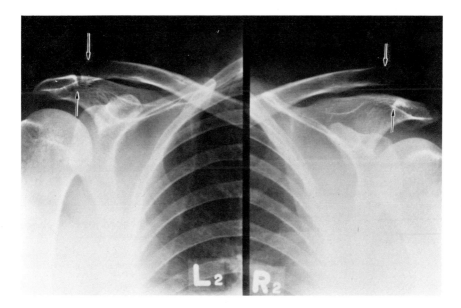

Fig. 5-10.
   Comparative views of both shoulders, showing separation of the right acromioclavicular joint. Notice the distance between the arrows on the right as compared to that on the left.

used to signify a decrease in bone density, regardless of the etiology; and in some textbooks, *osteopenia* is also used to describe the same changes.

   In order to produce bone, osteoid must be laid down, normally mineralized, and normally removed by physiological processes. A defect in osteoid production leads to osteoporosis; a defect in mineralization, osteomalacia; and a defect in removal of bone, osteolysis. The manner in which osteoid balance is maintained is rather complicated and is based primarily on a combination of dietary intake and absorption, hormonal interplay, and normal stress or muscular activity.

   Osteoporosis due to hormonal deficiency is quite common in postmenopausal women. Loss of bone density following trauma or nerve injuries (Sudeck's atrophy) occurs probably due to hyperemia following the trauma, with perhaps hormonal interplay superimposed. Thinning of bone also occurs in disease processes such as sickle cell anemia and other myelogenic osteopathies (Fig. 5-11).

Osteomyelitis. Osteomyelitis is by definition infection of the bone and bone marrow. In osteitis the bone, alone, is affected. Infection may be from pyogenic or nonpyogenic organisms, with the infection occurring either by direct extension from a wound or by hematogenous spread, especially originating from skin lesions. Infection results from a combination of low host resistance and virulence of the

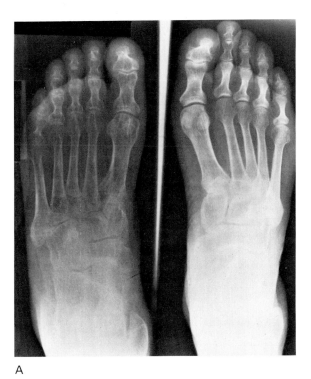

A

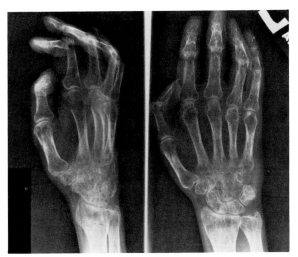

B

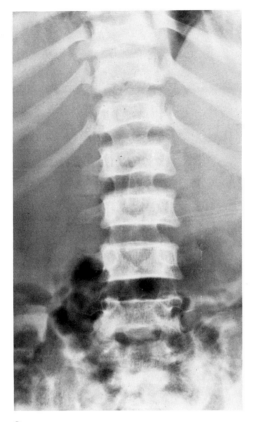

C

Fig. 5-11.
(A) Comparative views of the right and left feet, showing marked disuse osteoporosis of the left foot following an ankle injury. Notice how the trabecular pattern is more prominent in the osteoporosis as compared to the normal right foot.
(B) Marked osteoporosis of the hand (Sudeck's atrophy) following an elbow injury.
(C) Sickle cell anemia showing typical collapsed vertebrae. Changes similar to these may be seen in postmenopausal osteoporosis.

organism or either factor alone. Most osteomyelitis is caused by *Staphylococcus aureus,* with only a small proportion caused by streptococci, *Escherichia coli,* and *Neisseria gonorrhoeae.* Most infections involve the metaphyses of the bone, particularly at the end where most rapid growth occurs.

Roentgenographically, no change may be seen for the initial seven to ten days of the infection. Following this period of time, one may see a periosteal elevation, with osteolysis following early (Fig. 5-12). Associated with the bony reaction, soft tissue swelling may be present. As the process becomes chronic, the bone

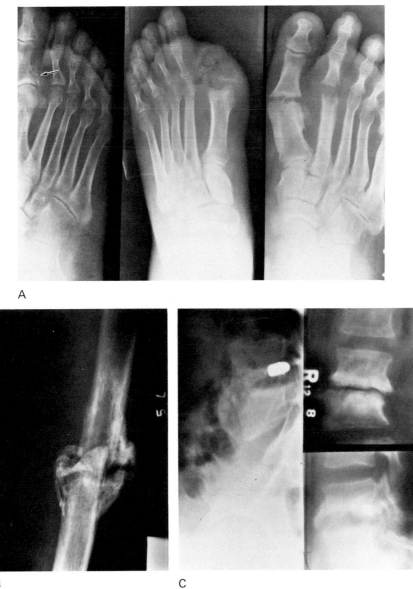

Fig. 5-12.

(A) Three typical cases of diabetic osteomyelitis demonstrating changes ranging from periosteal reaction to complete destruction of a phalanx.

(B) Chronic osteomyelitis involving a femoral fracture. Notice the bone destruction extending into the shaft and the marked periosteal reaction.

(C) Osteomyelitis involving the disk space following a gunshot wound. The disk space is narrowed, and there is sclerotic bone present. A mild subluxation is present.

dies and may present a sclerotic appearance about the osteolysis. New bone is formed which is variable and somewhat dependent upon the degree of severity of the infection. Since there must be approximately 50 percent of the bone destroyed before the disease can be appreciated roentgenographically, after the initial identification of osteomyelitis roentgenographic examinations are generally not very helpful in delineating the extent of the osteomyelitis and on occasion may not be helpful in determining recurrence of infection within a specific area.

Arthritis

By definition, arthritis refers to inflammation of a joint. In actual practice this is not always true, since there are many instances in which there are degenerative changes involving the joint but no etiological infective agent identifiable. Some years ago the term *rheumatism* was used to imply arthritis, and many patients today refer to arthritis as "rheumatism." There are a host of etiological factors for arthritis, including pyogenic, trauma, collagen disease, gout, and many others. Acute arthritis is marked by the presence of pain, heat, redness, and swelling about a joint. In many cases, arthritis is not present but arthralgia (joint pain) is noted. In acute arthritis sometimes the only way the diagnosis can be made is by examination of the joint fluid. In addition, as aging progresses there are certain degenerative changes involving the joint spaces which can only be described as degenerative joint disease.

Pyogenic Arthritis. This is generally secondary to staphylococcal, streptococcal, or gonococcal infections; and these infections usually respond rapidly to antibiotics. Generally, a focus of infection may be found elsewhere on the skin or within the body. The early roentgenographic changes show an increase in joint space with loss of bone density about the joint. As the disease continues, there is progressive loss of the joint space with destruction of the cartilage. Eventually there will be erosion and destruction of subarticular bone and, with further destruction, subluxation and dislocation of the joint (Fig. 5-13). As the process heals, there is recalcification, sclerosis, and ankylosis of the joint.

Tuberculous Arthritis. Tuberculous arthritis is seen only occasionally. Generally there is a focus of infection in the chest. Tuberculosis usually destroys articular cartilage and disks and generally does not show any prominent periosteal reaction or sequestrous sclerosis as noted in pyogenic osteomyelitis (Fig. 5-14). It is notable that changes occur much more slowly in tuberculosis than in pyogenic arthritis.

Rheumatoid Arthritis. Rheumatoid arthritis typically begins in the peripheral joints. The disease process also involves the distal ulna and styloid process of the ulna. Rheumatoid arthritis tends to be symmetrical and is classically

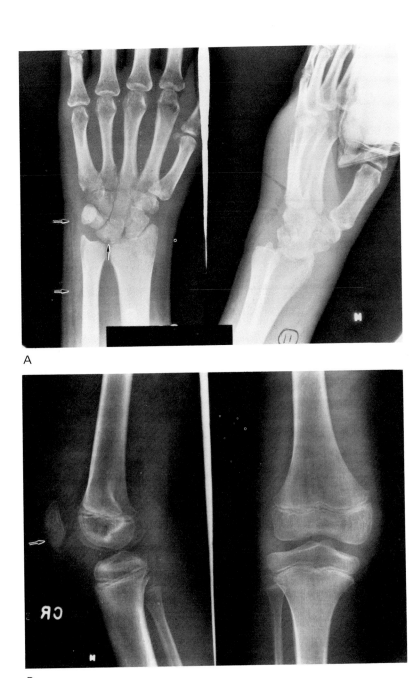

A

B

Fig. 5-13.

(A) Gonococcal arthritis of the wrist. Notice the air within the soft tissues and the bone destruction at the base of the lunate bone.

(B) Streptococcal arthritis of the knee. Notice the marked soft tissue swelling and the minor bone changes in the patella (arrow).

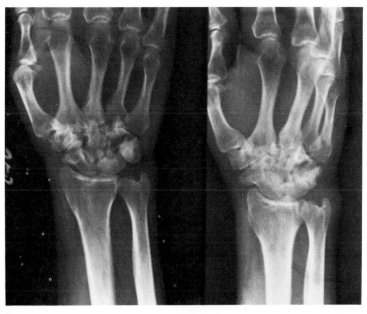

A

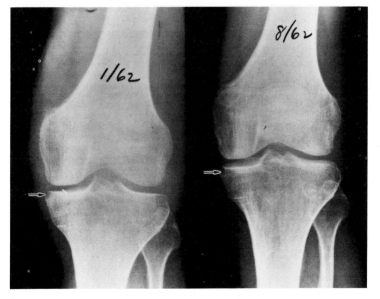

B

Fig. 5-14.

(A) Tuberculosis of the wrist. Notice the moth-eaten appearance of the carpals. The distal radius, ulna, and metacarpals are normal.

(B) Tuberculosis of the knee. Initially no roentgen signs were present. Bone changes occur late and involve the margins of the joint. Notice the pea-shaped defects in the cortical margins and the changes over a seven-month period.

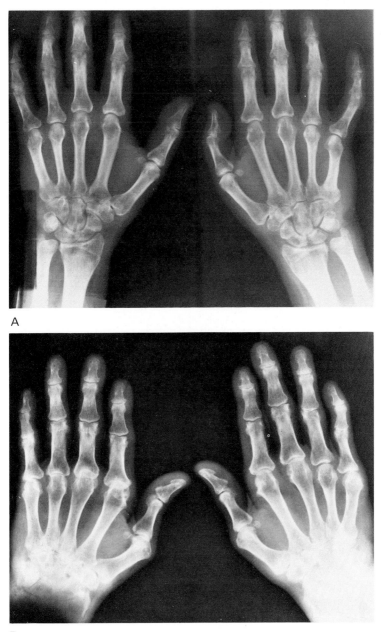

A

B

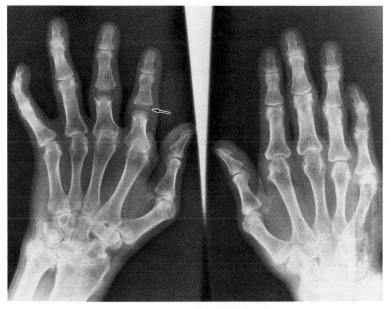

C

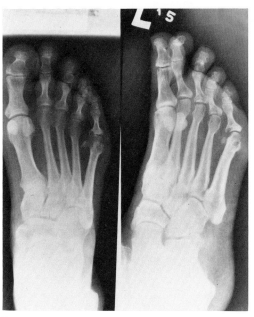

D

Fig. 5-15.
Rheumatoid arthritis. (A) Notice the periarticular changes involving the proximal inter-phalangeal joints. There are juxtaarticular erosions, osteoporosis, narrowing of the joint spaces, and soft tissue swelling about all the proximal interphalangeal joints.

(B) Marked soft tissue changes of rheumatoid arthritis. Several of the middle interpha-langeal joints have subluxation. (C) Same patient as (B) two years later and now with proximal interphalangeal prosthesis (arrow).

(D) Rheumatoid arthritis involving the foot. Note the changes at the MP joint of the fifth toe and compare to (A).

described as "waxing and waning." Rheumatoid arthritis is primarily a disease of the synovia, producing an extravasation of the vascular connective tissue termed a *pannus*. It more commonly affects women than men and is generally more often seen in the third and fourth decades of life. Rheumatoid arthritis is known by its many and diverse clinical appearances. It may present as an acute febrile illness with rapid destruction of joints or as one in which the manifestation is that of chronicity, with the patient never really having acute joint pain. On occasion, rheumatoid nodules may be felt in the subcutaneous tissue, particularly around the olecranon bursa.

Roentgenographically, the earliest signs are those of fusiform swelling about the involved joint. Focal juxtaarticular osteoporosis then occurs, and this is believed to be secondary to disuse osteoporosis and hyperemia. Marginal erosions occur which are caused by pressure from the pannus on the edges of the articular spaces. These may be very small but are quite significant roentgenographically. As the disease progresses, there is narrowing of the joint spaces secondary to degeneration of the articular cartilage. In the later stages, subluxations, contractions, and ankylosis occur (Fig. 5-15).

The above roentgenographic findings may also be seen in other collagen diseases such as systemic lupus erythematosis and scleroderma. Although the disease is primarily that of women in the third or fourth decade, it still may be seen in men and children.

Rheumatoid Spondylitis. This is essentially the same disease process as rheumatoid arthritis, but different etiological agents are suggested. Rheumatoid spondylitis generally involves the synovial joints of the spine and affects the male more often than the female. Roentgenographically, one initially sees bilateral blurring of the sacroiliac joints and squaring of the vertebral bodies (Fig. 5-16). If only one sacroiliac joint is involved, one should think of rheumatoid arthritis before rheumatoid spondylitis. The characteristic feature of the disease is bony ankylosis of the involved joints. Calcification of the spinal ligaments occurs which produces the characteristic bamboo appearance of the spine, or the so-called poker spine. Recently, involvement of the disk space has been described, and these changes are quite similar to those of tuberculosis or Pott's disease.

Gouty Arthritis. This arthritis is secondary to a metabolic error in the metabolism of the amino acid, purine. Elevated levels of uric acid may be secondary to the increased production of uric acid or due to the increased destruction of cells containing significant amounts of uric acid. Somewhat akin to rheumatoid arthritis, gout is characterized by acute attacks interwoven with intervals of symptom remission. It most often affects the metatarsophalangeal joint of the great toe, which has been clinically described as being swollen, tender, painful, and having a bluish red color (Fig. 5-17).

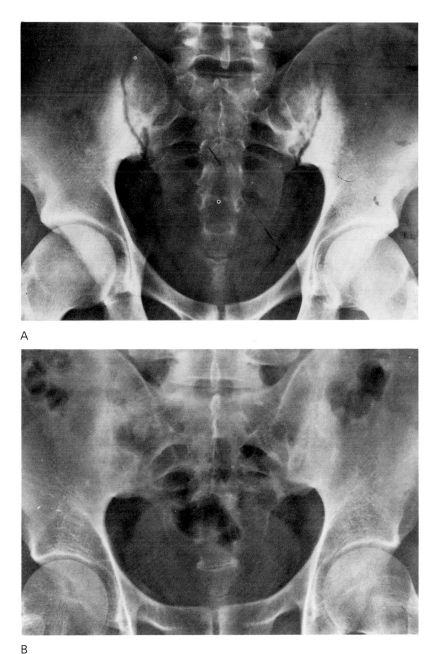

A

B
Fig. 5-16.
Rheumatoid spondylitis. (A) Early reactive changes involving the sacroiliac joints.
(B) Late changes, with the sacroiliac joints nearly obliterated.

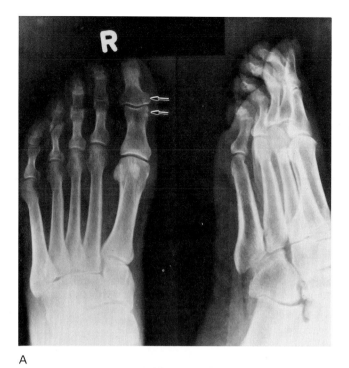

A

B

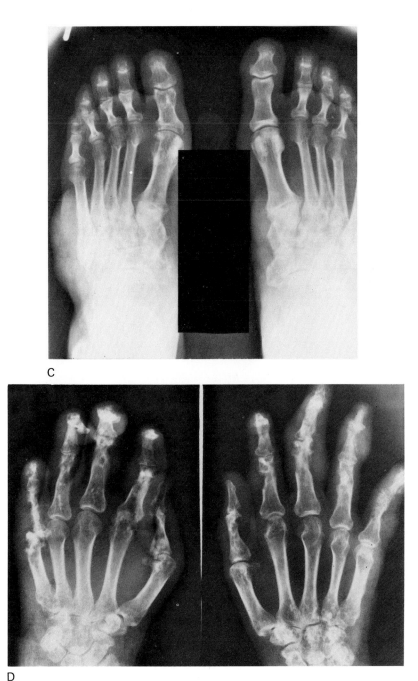

C

D

Fig. 5-17.
   Gouty arthritis. (A) Early changes, right great toe. The articular surface is intact; compare to Figure 5-16A. (B) Changes involving both great toes, with cystlike defects and soft tissue swelling. (C) Destruction of the tarsals, with large tophus along the lateral margin of the foot. (D) Severe destruction of the hand from gouty arthritis.

Roentgenographic changes occur late and are due to the deposition of sodium urate crystals adjacent to the joint space. Tophi appear as late changes and roentgenographically are seen as fairly well-defined cavities surrounded by thin, sclerotic walls. The tophi may be marginal, within the bone, or on occasion erode from soft tissue depositions.

In comparing gout and rheumatoid arthritis, it is noted that the erosion of the articular surfaces and loss of the joint space are much more common in rheumatoid arthritis and are seldom seen in gout.

Osteoarthritis (Degenerative Joint Disease, Hypertrophic Arthritis). This is generally a disease of older persons that affects the weight-bearing joints and interphalangeal joints of the fingers. The changes may occur primarily from aging or secondary to stress, strain, or trauma.

Roentgenographically, the highlight of degenerative joint disease is that of spurring, or the formation of osteophytes (Fig. 5-18). These begin on the articular edges of the bones and produce lipping of the joint space. As the

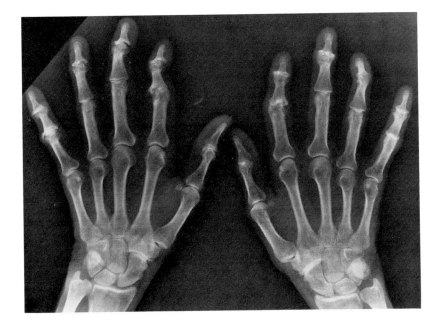

Fig. 5-18.

Osteoarthritis. Notice the spurring involving primarily the distal interphalangeal joints, with no involvement of the styloid process of the ulna. The styloid process is much more frequently involved with rheumatoid arthritis than it is with osteoarthritis.

process proceeds, eburnation or increased sclerotic density around the joint becomes more prominent, particularly about the large weight-bearing joints. There may be some decrease in joint space, but this is uneven as compared to the uniform destruction of the joint bone in rheumatoid arthritis. The degenerative joint space, particularly in the hips, sometimes presents cystic lesions with sclerotic rims. As the disease worsens, there may be subluxation of the joint; and loose calcific bodies may be seen within the joint space.

Bursitis. Although not an arthritis as purely defined, bursitis is included because of its connotation from the old name of rheumatism. Bursitis is a nonpyogenic inflammation of the bursae surrounding tendons, generally affecting the supraspinous tendon and found roentgenographically above the greater tuberosity of the humerus. About half the patients with bursitis have demonstrable calcific deposits within the tendon (Fig. 5-19). Also, on occasion bursitis may affect the greater trochanter of the femur. Occasionally one may see calcific deposits in tendons in asymptomatic patients.

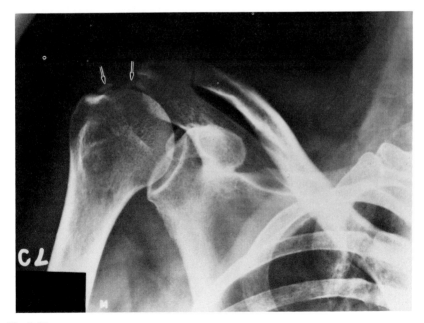

Fig. 5-19.
   Bursitis or peritendonitis calcarea. Notice the calcification just above the humeral head. Calcification such as this may be seen in asymptomatic patients.

NEOPLASTIC DISEASE OF BONE

Bone tumors are seen in patients of all ages. Most tumors can be identified by
roentgenographic means, but it is beyond the scope of this presentation to
present anything but the briefest outline of bone tumors. It is generally the
responsibility of the radiologist to determine whether a bone tumor is malignant or benign. By evaluating the patient's age, location of the tumor, pattern
of bone destruction, and its position within the bone, the radiologist may be
able to contribute a definitive diagnosis of the bony abnormality

Benign Bone Tumors

The most common benign tumor seen is a benign osteochondroma (Fig. 5-20).
This appears as an exostosis arising from the bony cortex and merging with the
spongiosa of the bone. It is capped by a rim of cartilage which is radiolucent;
but in older persons, this cartilage calcifies so that the entire tumor may be
identified. These are more commonly seen around the knee and proximal ends

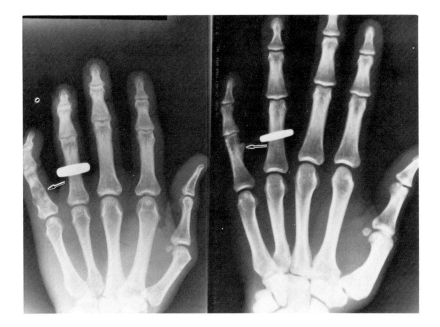

Fig. 5-20.
   Comparative films of an osteochondroma on the right and an enchondroma on the left
in different patients. Both lesions are benign tumors.

of the humerus. This tumor is generally asymptomatic except when it is involved with trauma.

Bone cysts are generally not clinically evident and are usually only noted when there is pain associated with increased growth of the cyst or when a pathological fracture occurs (see Fig. 5-6; Fig. 5-21). The etiology may be that of a simple bone cyst, but giant cell tumors, aneurysmal bone cysts, and eosinophilic granuloma must be included in the differential diagnosis.

Osteoid osteoma is another benign bone tumor; it occurs most frequently in children and young adults (Fig. 5-22). This tumor may be found in almost any bone in the body, and it characteristically presents as a focus of pain occurring most often at night which is almost completely relieved by aspirin. A roentgenogram will demonstrate an area of sclerosis within which is a radiolucent center termed a *nidus.* Sometimes the nidus is not identifiable but may be shown with tomograms.

Malignant Bone Tumors

These occur in patients of all ages. In the young child, the most common tumor is Ewing's sarcoma (Fig. 5-23), which may frequently be misdiagnosed as osteomyelitis.

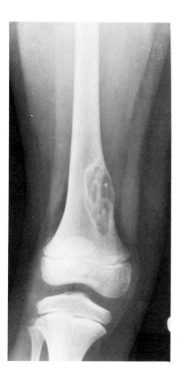

Fig. 5-21.

Cystic fibroxanthoma of the femur. The lesion shows no associated soft tissue mass, bone destruction, or periosteal reaction as is normally seen in malignant tumors.

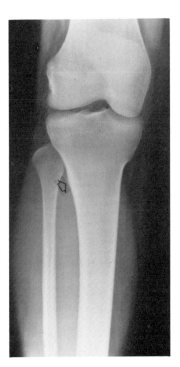

Fig. 5-22.

Osteoid osteoma. The only abnormality seen
is a sclerotic widening of the cortex at the arrow.
Osteoid osteomas are painful, are relieved by
aspirin, and are sometimes difficult to demonstrate
roentgenographically. A central nidus was demonstrated in this lesion by planigraphy.

Fig. 5-23.

Ewing's sarcoma involving the upper humerus.
Notice the moth-eaten appearance of the bone destruction, the marked periosteal reaction, and the soft tissue
mass associated with this malignant tumor.

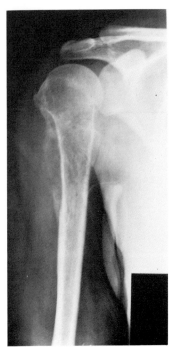

Osteogenic sarcoma, chondrosarcoma, and fibrosarcoma are the more common tumors arising from bone cartilage and fibrous tissue. These tumors occur in almost every age group, but chondrosarcoma is most commonly seen in older patients, as is fibrosarcoma. Osteogenic sarcoma is a tumor of the younger person (Fig. 5-24).

Constant low-grade pain is the predominant symptom of malignant bone tumors. By the time a definite mass is discernible and roentgenographic examination is made, the tumor most likely has progressed to the metastatic stage; and survival rates at this point are extremely discouraging.

Multiple Myeloma. Multiple myeloma is the most common primary tumor involving bone. It is so termed because of the appearance of multiple lesions within the bone which arise from the plasma cells of the bone marrow. Laboratory findings include an elevation of the globulin fraction of the blood protein and the appearance of Bence Jones protein within the urine. The punched-out lesions as have been described generally do not show sclerosis except under rather marked and heavy chemotherapy (Fig. 5-25).

Metastatic Bone Tumors. Unfortunately metastatic bone tumors may be the first sign of malignancy elsewhere in the body. This is particularly true of lung and renal tumors. Characteristically metastatic bone tumors are not relieved by rest and are aggravated by activity. Pathological fractures may occur; and on occasion, biopsy of the bone lesion may suggest the primary malignancy (Fig. 5-26).

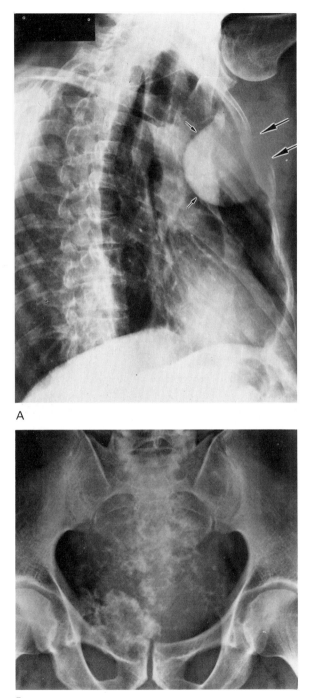

A

B

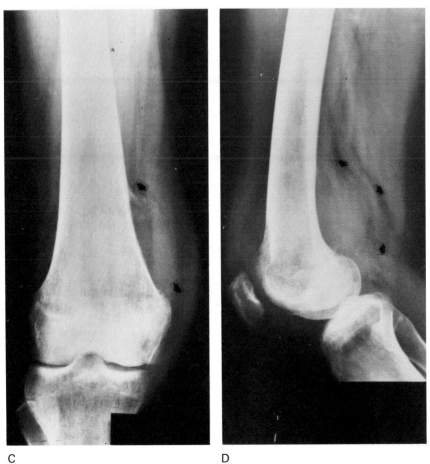

C   D

Fig. 5-24.

(A) Fibrosarcoma of the chest wall destroying the ribs.

(B) Chondrosarcoma of the pelvis. Notice the popcorn-type calcification extending from the right pubic ramus up into the pelvis. The upper margin of the ramus is destroyed by tumor.

(C) Osteogenic sarcoma showing a large tissue mass with a periosteal reaction. (D) Lateral view of (C).

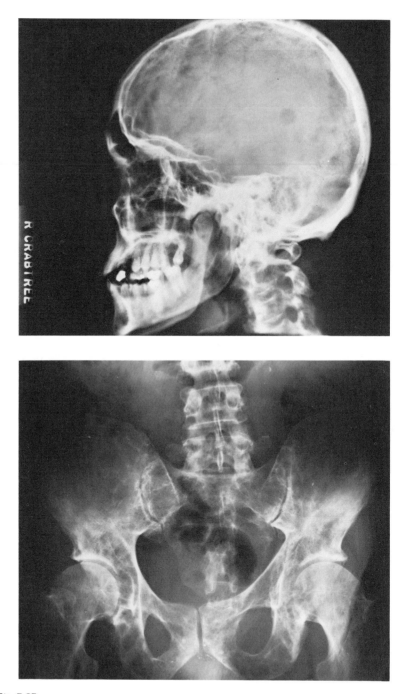

Fig. 5-25.
Multiple myeloma with typical punched-out lesions involving the skull and pelvis.

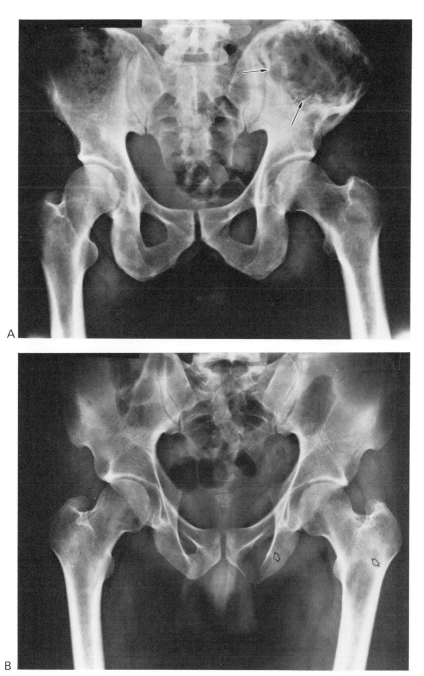

Fig. 5-26.
  Metastatic bone tumors. (A) Reticulum cell sarcoma metastatic to the left ilium.
(B) Undifferentiated sarcoma to the pelvis and left femur.

SPINAL PROBLEMS

In addition to the subjects discussed previously, perhaps back pain is one of the more common entities seen in a general medical setting. Although the bony skeleton may be involved in most of these etiologies, one should not forget that in the male one of the more common causes of back pain is disease involving the kidneys and, particularly, the prostate gland.

Disk disease is one of the most common causes of pain in the neck and low back. With degeneration of the disks, pain may be referred due to concomitant muscle spasm. One must differentiate between a so-called slipped disk and muscular ligamentous strain, which generally can be relieved by the injection of a topical anesthetic in the areas of maximum tenderness. Thoracic pain may be referred from a slipped cervical disk.

Low back pain is much more common than thoracic or cervical spine pain. Degenerative joint diseases may be evident in the lumbar area. Spurring or lipping of the lumbar spine does occur in asymptomatic patients, however, and the presence of such spurs does not indicate acute arthritis per se. Chronic low-grade back pain may be secondary to disarrangement of the articular facets of the lumbar vertebral bodies or to congenital anomalies (Fig. 5-27). One should also recognize that poor posture or the shortening of leg length may produce a stress on the lower lumbar area and cause constant pain. In addition, lack of sufficient arch within the metatarsals may also result in low back pain.

Spondylolysis with spondylolisthesis is a slippage of the vertebral bodies one upon another due to a defect in the pedicle. Although spondylolysis has been considered a congenital abnormality in the pars interarticularis of the vertebral body, it is now generally thought that most spondylolysis is secondary to an old fracture of the pars interarticularis. Depending upon the degree of slippage, spondylolisthesis is described roentgenographically as being first, second, or third degree (Fig. 5-28). Spondylolisthesis may have the same symptoms as a lumbar disk.

Herniated lumbar discs are commonly seen in general medical practice. Pain in the back may be acute and severe, radiating into one or both legs. The evaluation of herniated disc is done by myelography and will be described in Chapter 13, Special Procedures in Radiology.

In order to evaluate the spine, the PA (AP), lateral, and both oblique views must be obtained. In the cervical spine, spot films are also made of the odontoid process; and in the lumbar spine, a spot film is made of the L-5–S-1 interspace. For the thoracic spine, most radiologists believe that oblique views are confusing because of the overlying rib shadows that are projected over the spine.

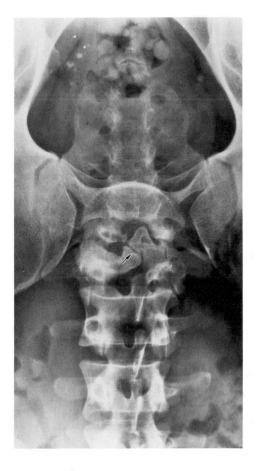

Fig. 5-27.
Spina bifida and lumbarization of S-1. These are congenital defects and are commonly seen in asymptomatic patients.

Back pain may also be secondary to referred pain from hip disease. In many instances, roentgenograms of the lumbosacral spine should also include a flat plate of the pelvis to demonstrate the hips. Figure 5-29 gives examples of different diseases of the hips.

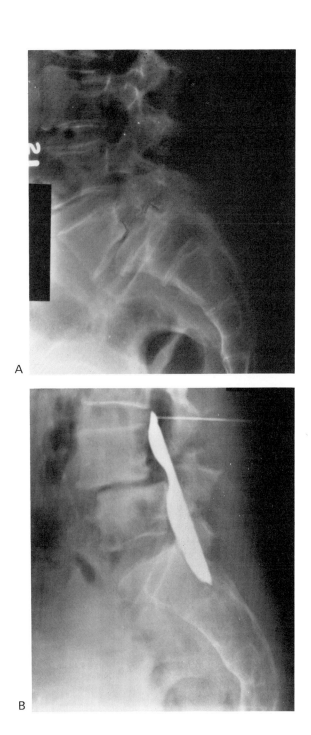

Fig. 5-28.

(A) Spondylolisthesis, second degree, L-5—S-1. The margins of the vertebral bodies are marked to indicate the degree of slippage. (B) Spondylolisthesis, L-4—L-5, with myelogram demonstrating pressure defect on spinal canal.

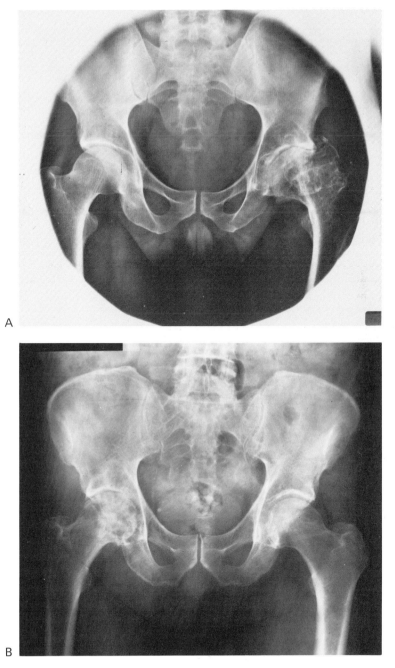

A

B

Fig. 5-29.

Common hip problems. (A) Traumatic arthritis, left hip, from war injury. The right hip is normal.

(B) Aseptic necrosis, both hips, worse on the right than on the left. The right hip joint is more narrowed than the left. Cystic destruction is apparent on the right and is demonstrated by tomograms on the left.

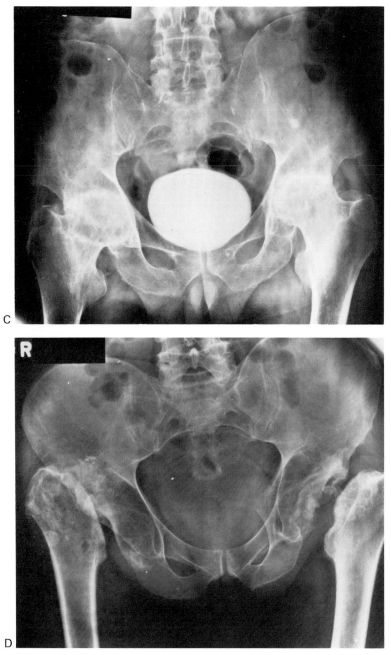

C

D

Fig. 5-29 (continued)

   (C) Rheumatoid arthritis. Both hip joints are involved; they are narrowed and partially destroyed.

   (D) Legg-Perthes' disease. There has been complete destruction with subluxation of both femoral heads.

READING LIST

Aegerter, E., and Kirkpatrick, J. A., Jr. *Orthopedic Diseases.* Philadelphia: Saunders, 1968.
Edeiken, J., and Hodes, P. J. *Roentgen Diagnosis of Diseases of Bone.* Baltimore: Williams
    & Wilkins, 1967.
Jaffe, H. L. *Tumors and Tumorous Conditions of the Bones and Joints.* Philadelphia: Lea
    & Febiger, 1958.

Plain Films of the Abdomen

6

THE ABDOMEN IS BOUNDED by the diaphragm above and the pelvis below, with the abdominal wall as its outer limit. In scanning the abdominal film, one should follow a particular pattern so as to visualize all structures. This pattern will vary from observer to observer, but a pattern is necessary to avoid a haphazard scanning method.

Renal Outlines (Fig. 6-1a). The kidney shadows are usually fairly well seen. They are grossly the same size, with smooth outlines and with the lower poles canted outward to about the same degree as the psoas shadows. Any calcific densities overlying the renal shadows should be noted.

Ureters (Fig. 6-1b). Follow the course of the ureters and note the presence of calculi in the region.

Psoas Stripes (Fig. 6-1c). These should be symmetrical. Retroperitoneal masses may obliterate a portion of a psoas stripe, and absence of a portion of the stripe should be noted. Old retroperitoneal infections may obliterate the stripe, so the absence does not necessarily mean that a mass is present. A bulging psoas shadow in a patient with back pain may be an indication of an abscess or hematoma.

Spleen (Fig. 6-1d). Normally the spleen is located in the left upper quadrant and is generally not seen roentgenographically unless it is enlarged.

Liver and Gallbladder (Fig. 6-1e). The liver is in the right upper quadrant, and the tip may be seen just below the costal margin. Calcified gallstones may be visualized as either faceted or round, laminated densities in the right upper quadrant.

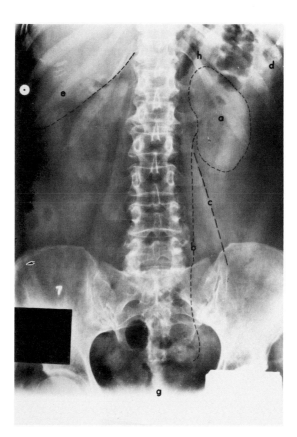

Fig. 6-1.
Plain abdominal film: a, renal outline; b, course of ureter; c, psoas stripe; d, region of spleen; e, region of liver and gallbladder; f, properitoneal fat stripe (arrow); g, urinary bladder; h, gastric air bubble.

Properitoneal Fat Stripes (Fig. 6-1f). This radiolucency extends from the costal margin down to the iliac crest and is easily separated from the abdominal musculature. The absence of this line may indicate peritoneal infection (peritonitis), flank abscess, appendicitis, or edema.

Intestinal Gas Pattern. The intestinal gas pattern is not only confusing to a novice but also may be so to an experienced radiologist. In infants and young children, it is common to see gas scattered throughout the bowel; but in the normal adult, gas is seen only in the stomach and colon. Unless the patient exhibits psychological aerophagy or is in pain, no appreciable gas should be seen in the small bowel. Hence, in most cases, the presence of small bowel gas indicates a pathological process.

Occasionally, particularly in a psychotic patient, aerophagy may be so pronounced that acute gastric dilatation may occur. This appears roentgenographically as an enlarged air and fluid-filled sac (Fig. 6-2). Jejunal obstruction may

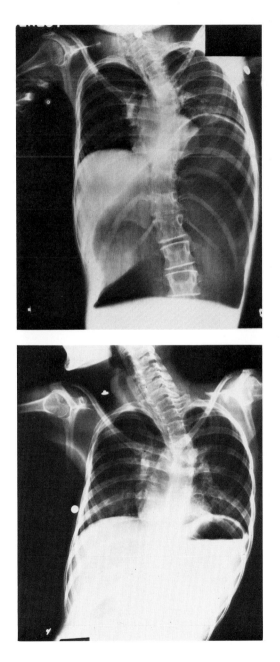

Fig. 6-2.
 Psychological aerophagy with acute gastric dilatation. This was a 12-year-old psychiatric patient. The bottom film was made twelve hours later.

be identified by its "coiled-spring" appearance (Fig. 6-3). Ileal obstruction may appear similar to colonic obstruction, but it lacks the haustral indentations and may present also as "stair-stepping" or layering of loops of bowel (Fig. 6-4). In some patients, obstructed loops may be so filled with fluid that large amounts of gas may not be demonstrable on flat abdominal films but may be readily seen on upright films (Fig. 6-5).

When one speaks of bowel obstruction, one generally refers to a paralytic or reflex ileus in which passage of bowel contents is prevented because of lack of normal peristalsis. In contrast, mechanical obstruction is due to actual compres-

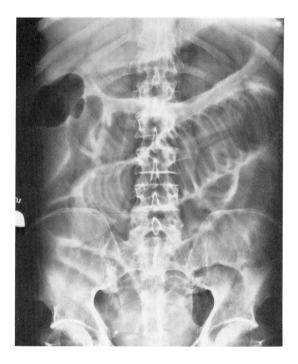

Fig. 6-3.

Small bowel obstruction secondary to carcinoma of the pancreas. Notice the typical "coiled-spring" appearance of the jejunum produced by distended valvulae conniventes. Compare to Figure 6-6.

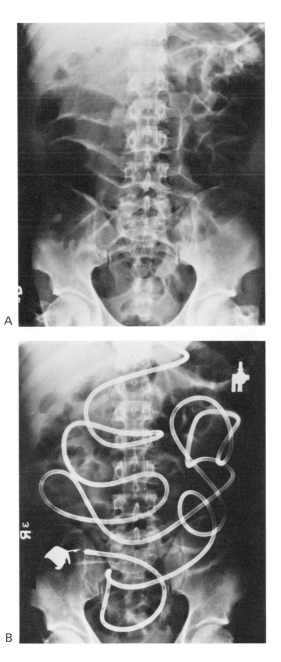

Fig. 6-4.

(A) Small bowel obstruction due to paralytic ileus secondary to carcinoma of the pancreas. Notice the "stair-stepping" of the ileum in the right abdomen. (B) Same patient decompressed by a Cantor tube.

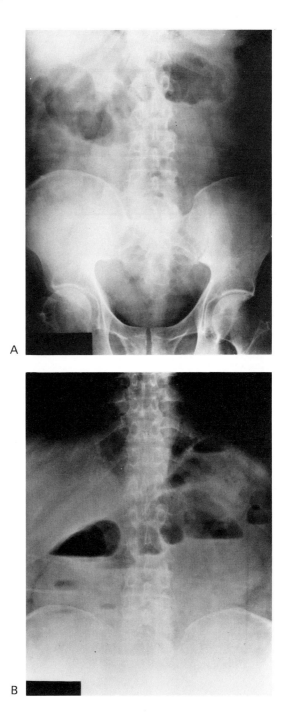

Fig. 6-5.

Small bowel infarction with perforation. (A) Flat plate showing the granular or ground glass appearance of ascites. (B) Upright abdominal film showing numerous air—fluid levels indicating obstruction, not appreciated on the flat plate. When looking for intestinal obstruction, it is almost mandatory that a lateral decubitus or upright film be obtained.

sion or blockage of the progression of bowel contents by mass lesion, adhesions, volvulus, or other impediments. There are gradations between each, and one may see a mild ileus with partial mechanical obstruction. Generally, distended bowel can be followed all the way to the rectum in ileus and may stop abruptly in mechanical obstruction. Localized ileus may produce the same signs as partial mechanical obstruction. On the upright films, air—fluid levels are not common in ileus and are quite common in mechanical obstruction. Greater distention in the small bowel occurs with mechanical obstruction than with ileus. An abnormally large amount of gas in the colon may suggest the presence of a volvulus (Fig. 6-6) or possibly a toxic megacolon from ulcerative colitis. On occasion, distention of the bowel is so marked that the level of obstruction is difficult to identify as being proximal colon or distal ileum (Fig. 6-7) or possibly distal colon (Fig. 6-8). Ascites, which is serous effusion into the abdominal cavity, may present a ground glass appearance of the abdomen.

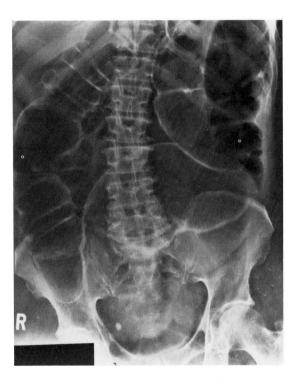

Fig. 6-6.
Sigmoid volvulus. Notice the marked amount of gas and the absence of haustral markings in the sigmoid colon, and compare this to the small bowel obstruction seen in Figure 6-7A. It is difficult at times to differentiate between large and small bowel obstruction.

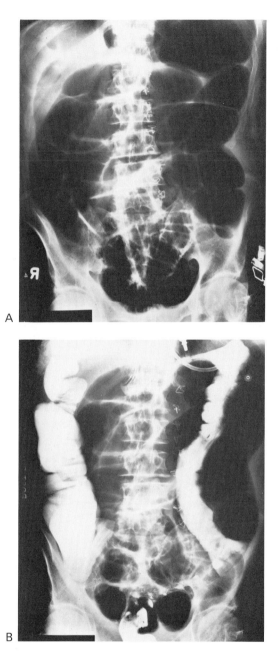

Fig. 6-7.
Small bowel obstruction secondary to adhesions following appendectomy. (A) Notice the marked distention of loops of small bowel. (B) Same patient. Barium enema demonstrates an obstruction at the terminal ileum.

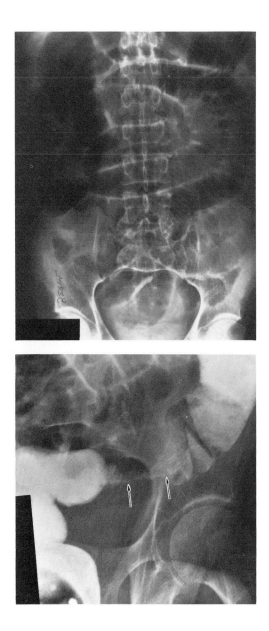

Fig. 6-8.
   Appearance of small bowel obstruction, but obstruction was found in the sigmoid colon. Acute sigmoid diverticulitis (arrows) was the cause of the obstruction.

Physical signs may be beneficial in differentiating ileus from mechanical obstruction. Absence of bowel sounds usually indicates ileus. Bowel rushes or "tinkles" may indicate mechanical obstruction. Vomitus containing bile indicates proximal small bowel obstruction. Paraumbilical pain indicates possible small rather than large bowel pathology. In evaluating such a patient, it may be beneficial to obtain a barium enema and reflux the barium retrograde up the small bowel to demonstrate an area of obstruction (see Fig. 6-7). Demonstration of mechanical obstruction usually indicates an emergency surgical procedure; whereas an ileus is usually treated medically.

Abdominal Mass. Plain films are also used for determining pathological entities within the abdomen. Calcification in the region of the pancreas suggests pancreatitis (Fig. 6-9). Localized calcification in the right upper quadrant suggests

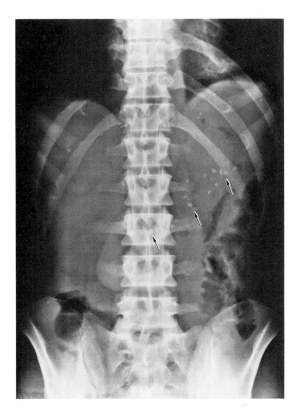

Fig. 6-9.
    Pancreatic calcification in the body of the pancreas. A normally opacified gallbladder is also seen.

gallstones, particularly if the calcification is laminated, faceted, or round (see Chapter 7). Renal stones overlie the kidneys and present as smooth or irregular densities. Irregular, popcorn-type calcifications may suggest necrotic tumor (Fig. 6-10). Gas outside the bowel may suggest perforation or an abscess (Fig. 6-11). Vascular calcification may be identified because of its curvilinear configuration (Fig. 6-12). Phleboliths in the pelvic veins can usually be identified because of their radiolucent centers. The localization of abdominal masses may also suggest an etiology; for example, a mass in the region of the spleen suggests splenic enlargement, disease involving the tail of the pancreas, or possibly a gastric mass. Displacement of normal bowel gas suggests the presence of a mass lesion, although the lesion itself may not be seen.

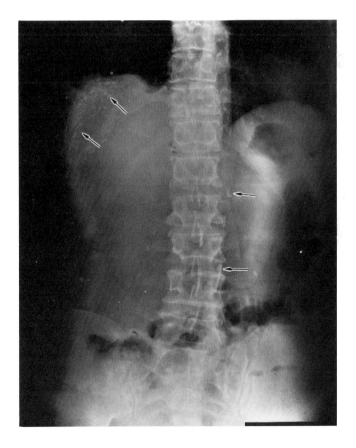

Fig. 6-10.
Metastatic carcinoma of the liver from the cecum. The calcification is due to necrotic tumor. Aortic calcification is noted to the left of the vertebral column.

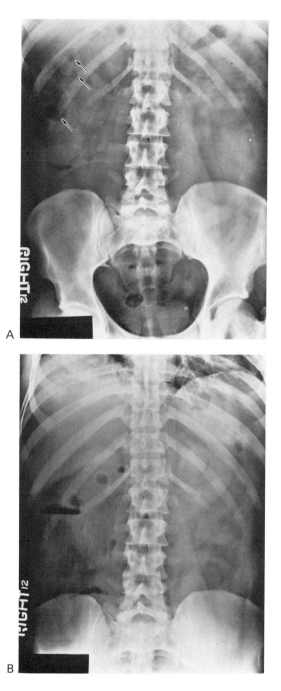

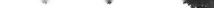

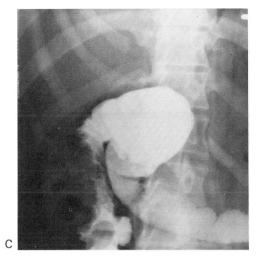

C

Fig. 6-11.

Subhepatic abscess secondary to ruptured appendix. (A) Flat plate. The gas pattern in the right upper quadrant suggests air outside the bowel. (B) Upright abdominal film. Notice the air—fluid level in the same area. (C) Barium enema demonstrating inflammatory changes of the colonic mucosa with numerous air bubbles in the adjacent abscess. Following drainage of the abscess and recuperation, the colon became entirely normal.

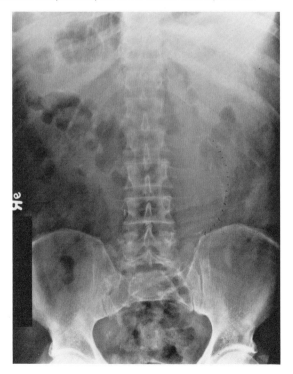

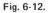

Fig. 6-12.

Abdominal aortic aneurysm. Notice the typical curvilinear vascular calcification.

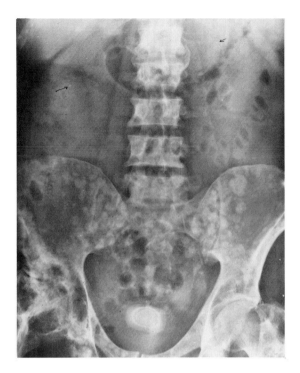

Fig. 6-13.
   Plain abdominal film taken for vague abdominal pain shows small renal stones (arrows),
a large laminated bladder stone, and widespread bony metastases from carcinoma of the
prostate gland.

Bony Structures. As has been described in the chapter on osseous anatomy, the
bones should be perused for any sign of misalignment, anomaly, or destruction.
On occasion, a kidney, ureter, and bladder film study taken for one reason may
demonstrate significant pathology elsewhere (Fig. 6-13).
   Plain films of the abdomen should be the initial roentgenographic examination
obtained in the evaluation of a patient presenting with or suspected of having
abdominal pain or other pathology. For more significant detail in examining
the abdomen, the student is referred to the major texts listed at the end of
Chapter 1.

The Biliary System

7

THE BILIARY SYSTEM (Fig. 7-1) is composed of the liver, gallbladder, and biliary tree. The liver occupies the upper right quadrant of the abdomen and may vary anatomically in size and shape. Systemic blood flow is from the hepatic artery, usually originating from the celiac axis. The portal vein transports nutrients from the bowel to the liver and then from the liver through the hepatic veins to the inferior vena cava. From the liver, right and left hepatic ducts arise to form the common bile duct, joined in its midportion by the cystic duct of the gallbladder. The common bile duct then courses posteriorly, ending on the medial posterior portion of the second portion of the duodenal loop at the ampulla of Vater. The orifice of the distal common duct is controlled by the sphincter of Oddi, located within the substance of the ampulla of Vater.

The Gallbladder. This organ is a pear-shaped sac located on the undersurface of the right lobe of the liver. The size of the gallbladder varies, but it is generally 7 to 10 cm in length and holds approximately one ounce of bile. Its wall is very thin, measuring only 1 to 2 mm; but in response to inflammation, it may become as much as several centimeters thick. The function of the gallbladder is to store and concentrate bile. Physiologically, there is very little hepatic bile produced until the liver is stimulated by the presence of food in the stomach. With food ingestion, bile is produced and flows through the hepatic ducts. Depending upon whether the sphincter of Oddi is closed or not, the bile is then forced through the cystic duct into the gallbladder, where it is stored; or if the pressure in the distal common duct is less than that of the cystic duct, the bile will flow through the common duct and into the duodenum. The cystic duct has numerous valves formed in the manner of a spiral which prevent emptying of the gallbladder until it has been stimulated by the presence of a cholecystokinin, which is released by the presence of fatty foods within the stomach. Generally, the gallbladder will concentrate to approximately one-tenth in volume the material entering its sac.

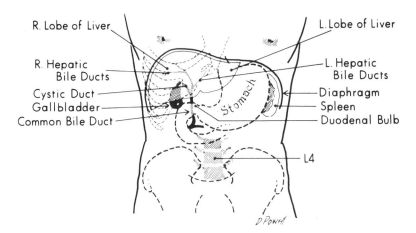

Fig. 7-1.
Anatomical relationships within the bile system: liver, bile ducts, and gallbladder.

There are many components of bile, and the gallbladder does not concentrate any component to the same degree.

Biliary Tree. Clinical symptoms peculiar to the biliary tract are pain and jaundice. Biliary colic is a misnomer, since biliary pain is sharp, boring, and continuous, rising to a crescendo and gradually diminishing to a dull ache. *Colic* refers to crampy or gripping-type pain that alternately increases and decreases in severity. The uniqueness of biliary pain is the point to which it radiates. If the pain originates in the hepatic or upper common duct, it refers directly to the right infrascapular area. If the gallbladder, cystic duct, or lower common duct are affected, the pain occurs in the right epigastric area and then radiates along the costal margin to the right scapula.

The presence of jaundice infers biliary stasis and regurgitation of bile back into the bloodstream. It is categorized into medical (nonobstructive) or surgical (obstructive) jaundice. Viral, toxic, and chemical hepatitis and hepatic cirrhosis are the more common causes of medical jaundice. Surgical jaundice may occur secondary to common duct obstruction, either by gallstones, carcinoma, or strictures resulting from scarring. Surgical jaundice usually presents slower than medical jaundice and also has less fever, leukocytosis, and pain than its medical counterpart. The serum alkaline phosphatase is generally higher in obstruction, whereas the thymol turbidity and serum glutamic oxaloacetic transaminase are higher in medical jaundice. The serum bilirubin is generally much higher in surgical jaundice than it is in medical jaundice. It is extremely important to recognize and differentiate medical from surgical jaundice, since surgery should be avoided in acute viral hepatic or acute pancreatic infections. Visualization of the biliary system with serum bilirubin up to 2 mg. per 100 ml. may be satisfactorily obtained with oral studies. With the bilirubin level above 2 mg. per 100 ml., visualization is poor and not seen at all in the presence of bilirubin above 4 mg. per 100 ml. The student should take the serum bilirubin level into consideration when requesting biliary tract examinations.

Gallstones are frequently demonstrated in persons with disorders of the biliary tract. Some 10 percent of the population may have gallstones, but only half of these patients will be symptomatic. In a patient with vague abdominal complaints, a gallbladder x-ray series may be helpful in ascertaining the etiology, since the presence of gallstones may infer biliary tract disease. One should also be aware that acute duodenal ulcers, myocardial infarction, right lower lobe pneumonia, hiatal hernias, and pleurodynia may mimic acute biliary tract disease; and these should be considered before proceeding to surgical exploration.

Plain films of the abdomen should be obtained preliminary to the introduction of any contrast media. The preliminary films may be necessary as a baseline, since faint calcifications may be obscured by the contrast material. In addition, these plain films may demonstrate pathology removed from the biliary system which could possibly preclude an examination of the biliary tree.

The Liver. This organ normally appears as a uniform soft-tissue density in the right upper quadrant. The size and shape may vary considerably, and a dozen different primary forms have been demonstrated by radioactive imaging. The diaphragm is the upper limit of the liver, although the lower posterior portion of the lung normally projects over the liver silhouette; it is normal to see pulmonary vessels projecting over the liver silhouette. The lower border of the liver usually conforms to the lower costal margin.

Hepatic enlargement occurs secondary to right heart disease or failure, hepatitis, early nutritional cirrhosis, primary and secondary neoplasias, and pyogenic or protozoan infections. Calcification is uncommon in general practice, although calcified hydatid cysts and lymph nodes may be seen on occasion. Air in the bile ducts is usually secondary to gas-forming pathogens or a fistula between the bile ducts and intestine, usually resulting from surgery or erosive carcinoma involving the ampulla of Vater and creating an incompetent common duct valve.

ROENTGENOGRAPHIC EXAMINATION OF THE GALLBLADDER

Examination of the gallbladder by contrast media is one of the more common studies in radiology. Gallstones may be recognized on a plain film of the abdomen (Fig. 7-2) as round densities which vary according to the amount of calcium salts within the stone. The more dense stones are usually calcium carbonate in content, with pure cholesterol or bile pigment stones generally invisible without

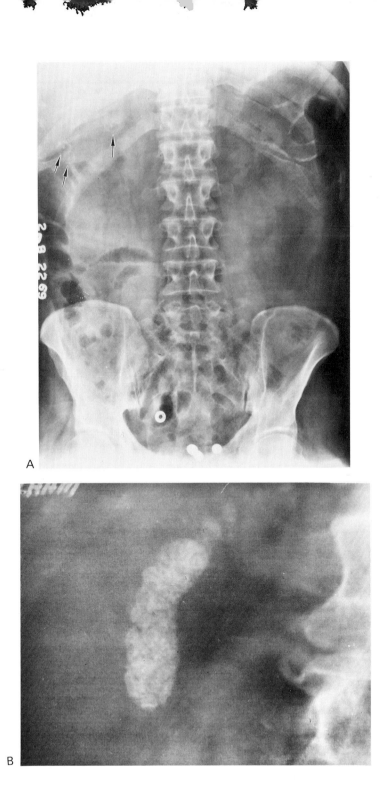

A

B

118

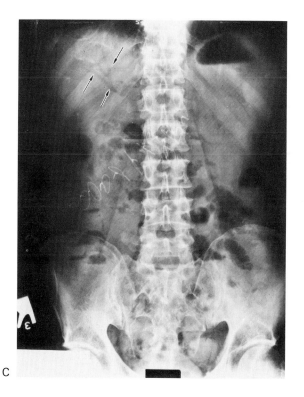

C

Fig. 7-2.
(A) Plain abdominal film. Note the laminated stones in the right upper quadrant overlying the liver. (B) Oblique film of the right upper quadrant showing a calcified gallbladder. (C) Plain film showing gas in the biliary tract which was later found to be secondary to a choledochoduodenostomy.

the aid of contrast material. If gallstones are demonstrated on the plain x-ray film, the value of a gallbladder examination would be to demonstrate the presence or absence of stones within the common bile duct. On occasion, differentiation between renal and biliary calculi from other calcifications must be made.

Successful demonstration of the gallbladder depends upon several factors. One of the more common causes of failure to visualize the gallbladder is the lack of absorption of the contrast material from the bowel. In patients with rapid transit of bowel contents, for example, from diarrhea, the contrast material may not be in the bowel long enough for absorption to occur. A technical factor is inadequate patient preparation. As has been mentioned previously, proper preparation of the patient for examination of the gallbladder is very important for the success of the study. If, for example, the patient is given a meal containing fat the night before the study, the gallbladder will be emptied and there will be an insufficient amount of contrast material stored in the gallbladder for adequate visualization. Lack of proper visualization may also be related to decreased secretion of bile from the liver secondary to liver disease.

Pathologically, the most common cause of nonvisualization of the gallbladder is obstruction of the cystic duct secondary to inflammation. On occasion, the cystic duct may be patent; but due to disease within the gallbladder wall, there is an inability of the gallbladder mucosa to concentrate the contrast media. Thus, visualization may be poor or nonexistent.

There are two drugs commonly used for examination of the gallbladder. Telepaque (iopanoic acid, U.S.P.) depends upon the concentrating ability of the gallbladder mucosa for visualization. The presence of chronic disease, obstruction of the cystic duct, or inadequate bile flow would cause poor or nonvisualization of the gallbladder. With the use of Oragrafin (calcium or sodium ipodate), there may be visualization in the presence of chronic disease of the gallbladder wall, since adequate visualization of the gallbladder does not depend upon the concentrating ability of the gallbladder wall but rather on the rapid absorption of the drug, normal bile flow, and patency of the cystic duct.

With failure of orally administered contrast media to visualize the gallbladder, intravenous cholangiography may be attempted (Figs. 7-3 and 7-4). It should be stated at the outset that examination by this means is rather tedious and time-consuming and may require the presence of the patient in the x-ray department for four hours or more. In addition, the contrast material may mix poorly with the bile and cause layering (Fig. 7-5) which may somewhat resemble floating gallstones. Toxic reactions are much more common and much more lethal with intravenous than with the oral method of administering contrast media.

The presence of rising serum bilirubin and alkaline phosphatase concentrations, which indicate obstruction of the common bile duct, may necessitate the

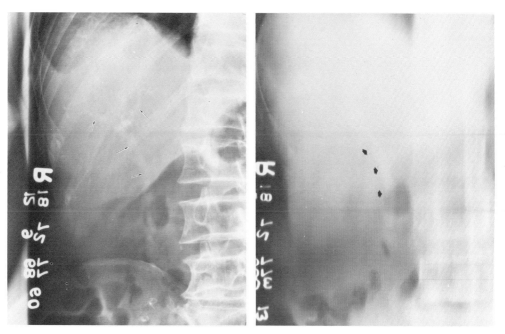

A   B

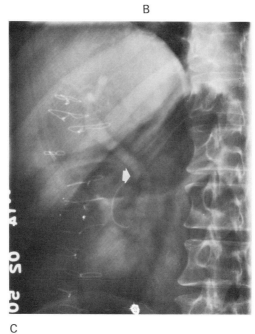

C

Fig. 7-3.

    (A) Normal intravenous cholangiogram. (B) Same patient as (A). This tomogram demonstrates the distal common duct more clearly. (C) Intravenous cholangiogram showing cystic duct remnant (arrow). The common duct is demonstrated well without tomography.

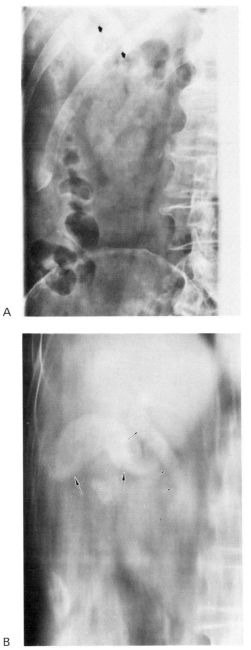

A

B

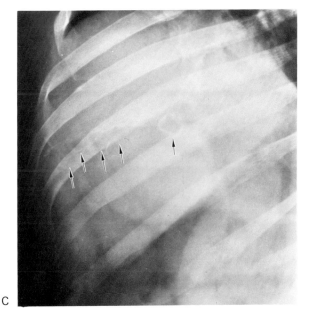

C

Fig. 7-4.

(A, B) A 75-year-old patient with signs and symptoms of cholecystitis. Initially the biliary system was not visualized by intravenous cholangiography. Repeat examination one month later shows poor visualization. Tomograms clearly delineate numerous radiolucent gallbladder (large arrows) and common duct stones (small arrows).

(C) A 45-year-old patient with intermittent right upper quadrant pain. Stones are well visualized, and all were in the right hepatic duct at operation.

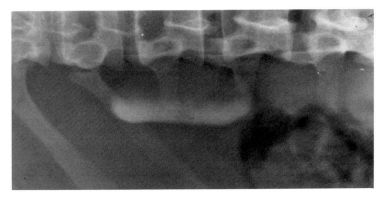

Fig. 7-5.

Layering of contrast media demonstrated on a lateral decubitus film following intravenous cholangiography.

performance of a percutaneous cholangiogram. Basically, the procedure involves inserting a needle into the biliary tree, withdrawing some of the bile, and instilling soluble contrast material in its place. This procedure is particularly helpful in evaluation of the distal common duct for the presence of stones or tumor involving the ampulla of Vater or the head of the pancreas (see Chapter 8).

Frequently during and following operation, soluble contrast media may be injected through a T tube to demonstrate patency of the common duct and to make certain that all stones have been removed. On occasion, a stone may be missed at operation, migrate to the distal common duct, and occlude bile passage into the duodenum (Fig. 7-6).

Having previously noted that a gallbladder examination is a common procedure in radiology, it should also be noted that the incidental finding of gallstones may not be an indication for operation. The clinical status of the patient, including findings referable to other diseases and his general physical condition, must all be taken into account in evaluation for an elective cholecystectomy.

Figures 7-7, 7-8, and 7-9 are representative examples of gallbladder examinations.

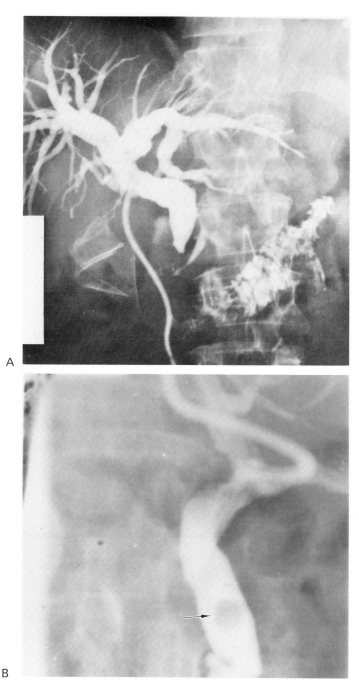

A

B

Fig. 7-6.

(A) T-tube cholangiogram. The changes in the distal common duct are inflammatory but may easily be confused with carcinomatous invasion. Note the reflux up the pancreatic duct.

(B) Spot film from postoperative T-tube cholangiogram. Note the radiolucent gallstone missed at surgery. Some of these stones may be dissolved with chemicals. One must be careful not to confuse a gas bubble for a radiolucent stone. Normally several spot films are made while contrast material is injected through the T-tube, during which time a gas bubble will change position whereas a gallstone will usually remain stationary.

125

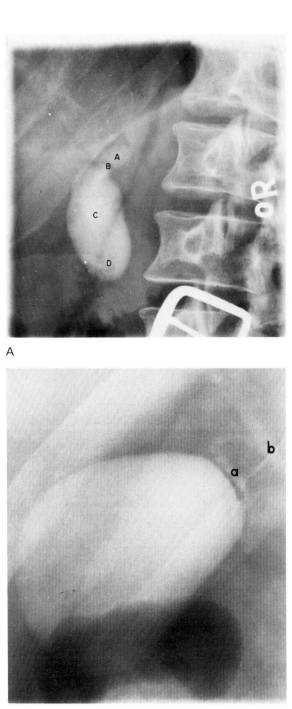

A

B

126

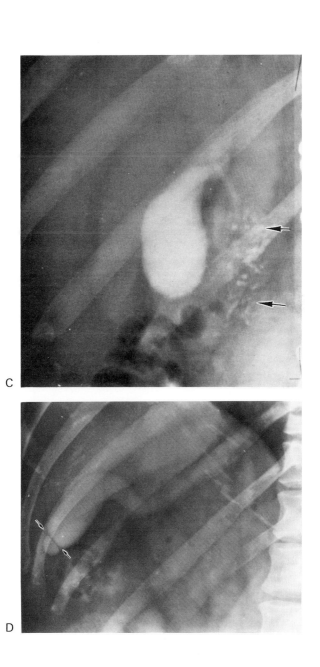

C

D

Fig. 7-7.

Normal gallbladder series. (A) Gross anatomy: A, neck; B, infundibulum; C, body; D, fundus of gallbladder.

(B) After stimulation of gallbladder by having the patient drink cream. The contracting gallbladder is emptying contrast material through a cystic duct (a) and the common duct (b).

(C) Normal gallbladder. Notice the calcium in the head of the pancreas.

(D) Gallbladder film demonstrating a septum through the fundus. This is normal and is called a *phrygian cap.*

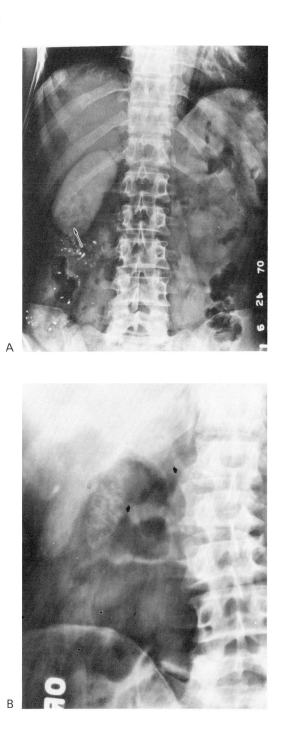

A

B

128

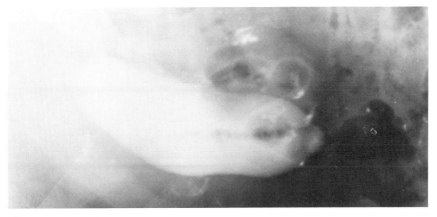

C

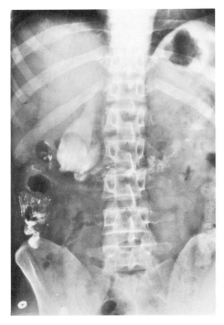

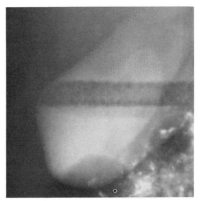

D   E

Fig. 7-8.

Cholelithiasis. (A) Numerous large radiolucent gallstones. (B) Asymptomatic 62-year-old patient with numerous gallbladder and common duct stones. (C) Layering of radiolucent stones on decubitus film.

(D) Routine anteroposterior scout film for gallbladder series. (E) Grossly normal, but upright film shows numerous small radiolucent stones. This is a good example of why a gallbladder series must consist of AP films plus a lateral decubitus or upright spot films.

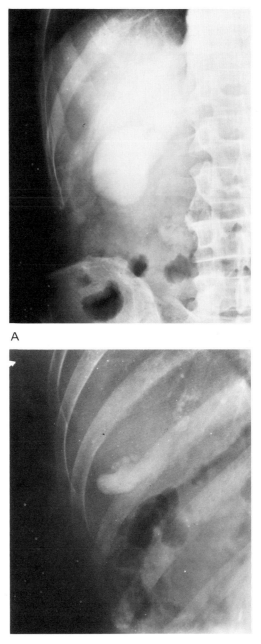

A

B

Fig. 7-9.

(A) Opacified gallbladder on an oral study demonstrating marked common duct dilatation secondary to carcinoma of the head of the pancreas.

(B) Adenomyosis of the gallbladder. Small stones were faintly seen on the original roentgenogram. Symptoms from adenomyomatosis may be similar to those of biliary or gallbladder dysfunction.

READING LIST

General

Wise, R. E. *Intravenous Cholangiography.* Springfield, Ill.: Thomas, 1962.

Specific

Wise, R. E. (Ed.). The Biliary System. *Radiol. Clin. North Am.* vol. 4, no. 3, 1966.
Wise, R. E. (Ed.). Radiology of the Liver, Biliary Tract, and Pancreas. *Radiol. Clin. North Am.* vol. 8, no. 1, 1970.

The Gastrointestinal Tract ⑧

DISEASES involving the gastrointestinal tract are as varied as diseases of the chest. Since our purpose in this text is to delineate normal from abnormal, only common occurrences will be described. Diseases and other conditions affecting the oropharynx and hypopharynx are relatively complicated and will not be included in this presentation.

Barium sulfate is the agent of choice for examination of the alimentary tract. Barium is inert and isotonic. Only two rules need to be applied in its use: (1) free passage through the colon must be certain; and (2) barium studies in a patient with suspected perforation of a hollow viscus must be approached with caution. Water-soluble contrast materials are useful on some occasions, but these agents are hypertonic and should be used with care in elderly or dehydrated patients and in the very young.

ESOPHAGUS

The esophagus is a muscular canal approximately 30 cm in length, extending from the posterior pharynx to the stomach. Its upper portion is at the level of C-6, and the gastroesophageal junction is at T-11. The upper esophagus is in the midline, but it swings slightly to the left as it courses behind and is indented by the aortic arch. Another indentation in the esophagus is noted at the level of the left main-stem bronchus, and there is another narrowing at the gastro-esophageal junction.

The esophagus also tends to follow the curvature of the dorsal spine and the course of the thoracic aorta. It is common to see the esophagus course poste-riorly with the development of an aging kyphosis. It is also common to see a tortuous esophagus relating to a tortuous aorta.

Food is propelled through the esophagus by a complex mechanism of propulsive and contractile peristalsis. In older patients and sometimes in patients with hiatal hernias, there is an asynchrony of the peristalsis resulting in what are termed *tertiary contractions* (commonly called *curling* or *corkscrew esophagus* (Fig. 8-1).

There are numerous disorders of the esophagus, including functional problems of spasm and achalasia. Entities such as diverticula, stricture, and tumors are also seen. Roentgenographic examination of the esophagus is performed by giving the patient small drinks of barium sulfate while he is being viewed with the fluoroscope. Overhead films are obtained of the barium filled esophagus at the discretion of the radiologist.

Esophageal Spasm and Achalasia. The main symptoms relating to esophageal spasm are intermittent difficulty in swallowing and substernal pain of varying degree. Roentgenographically, the esophagus may be perfectly normal, since

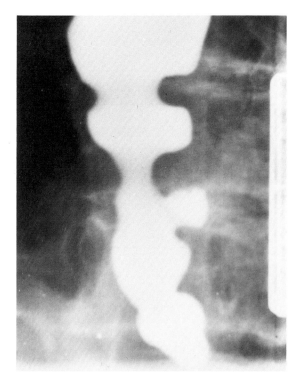

Fig. 8-1.

Tertiary contractions of the esophagus. Notice the corkscrew appearance. This is a benign condition seen in older patients and occasionally in patients with hiatal hernias.

spasm usually is of a transitory nature. Occasionally an intrinsic factor such as a tumor may be demonstrated.

Achalasia (Fig. 8-2), also known as cardiospasm and megaesophagus, is a dysfunction of peristalsis, with the defect noted at the gastroesophageal junction. Symptoms consist of heartburn, pain, dysphagia, and, occasionally, a sensation of food sticking at the level of the lower sternum or symptoms of esophageal overflow. Roentgenographically, the hallmark of achalasia is dilatation of the esophagus with a normal esophageal diameter noted at the gastroesophageal junction. The distal esophagus presents a typical beaking appearance which is the sine qua non for roentgenographic identification of achalasia. Differentiation must be made from carcinoma and benign strictures, but usually this is no problem.

Foreign Bodies (Fig. 8-3). These generally become lodged within the esophagus because of unintentional swallowing of a foreign body or lodging of a food particle because of poor mastication. Generally the patient is aware that a foreign body has been swallowed. He may be asymptomatic or may complain of pain and substernal burning, particularly on swallowing. Radiopaque foreign bodies are easily demonstrated, and PA and lateral films of the esophagus are usually sufficient to demonstrate them. Nonopaque foreign bodies are another matter, particularly chicken bones. Small slivers of bone may become embedded in the mucosa, producing pain on swallowing and occasionally causing perforation of

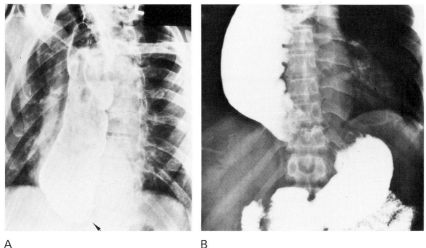

A   B

Fig. 8-2.
Achalasia. (A) Left anterior oblique view. Notice the dilated esophagus filled with barium and food particles. An arrow points to the so-called beaking seen in achalasia. (B) Same patient after colon interposition.

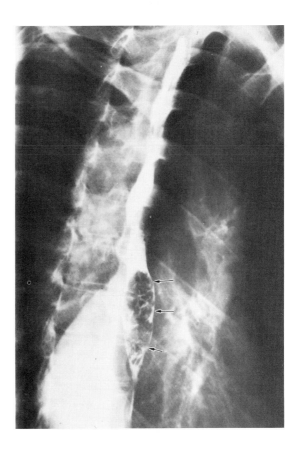

Fig. 8-3.
Foreign body in esophagus. Notice the large radiolucent filling defect in the lower esophagus. This foreign body was a piece of steak swallowed two days previously.

the esophagus with secondary mediastinitis or abscess formation. The nature of the foreign body should be indicated on the roentgenographic request form so that appropriate steps can be taken to demonstrate it.

Strictures (Fig. 8-4). These occur in many degrees, with symptoms varying according to the degree of obstruction. The patient may be asymptomatic initially and then slowly develops symptoms of food sticking, first solids and then liquids. Some strictures may become manifest after the patient receives his first pair of dentures or after extraction of a number of his own teeth with resultant poor mastication.

Strictures may occur secondary to ingestion of caustic material or reflux of

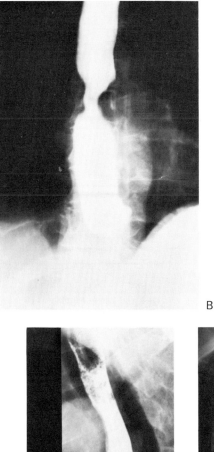

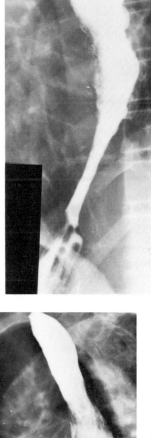

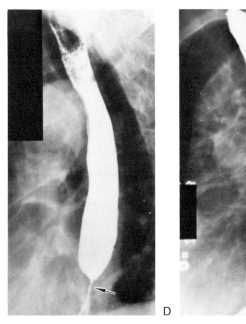

A

B

C

D

Fig. 8-4.

(A) Stricture of midesophagus of unknown etiology. It was surgically resected.

(B) Long stricture of distal esophagus secondary to prolonged gastric intubation. Notice the esophageal dilatation proximal to the stricture, typical of that found in benign lesions.

(C) Tight stricture of distal esophagus secondary to gastric reflux and esophagitis.

(D) Tight stricture following resection of distal esophagus and resultant gastric reflux (small arrow). Gastric mucosa is noted at the large arrow.

gastric contents from the stomach into the lower esophagus. A nasogastric tube left in the esophagus for a prolonged period of time may also create a persistent stricture. These strictures occur due to inflammation of the mucosa with resultant scarring of the entire thickness of the esophagus.

Roentgenographically, benign strictures generally show a dilatated esophagus proximal to the stricture in contrast to malignant strictures, which do not commonly have such a dilatation. Benign strictures may occur in a localized area or may extend over a large portion of the esophagus. The mucosa in the region of the stricture usually appears normal, and there is no abrupt change in the contour of the stricture as there is in malignant tumors.

Tumors. Malignant and benign tumors occur in the esophagus. Malignant tumors (Fig. 8-5) of the upper esophagus are usually squamous cell carcinoma. Tumors of the extreme lower esophagus may be either primary squamous cell carcinoma or adenocarcinoma invading from the stomach. Tumors of the lower third are more common than tumors of the upper or middle third of the esophagus. Benign tumors are almost always leiomyomata and are characterized by radiolucent intramural filling defects of the barium-outlined wall of the esophagus (Fig. 8-6).

Clinical symptoms vary according to the extent and severity of the obstruction secondary to the tumor. The first symptom is progressive dysphagia of short duration. Pain is uncommon, and when present it usually signifies extension of the tumor through the esophageal wall. Malignant tumors occur more often in males than in females and usually appear after the age of 40. Roentgenographically, the hallmark of malignant tumors is destruction of mucosa with ulceration. There is a sharp demarcation shown roentgenographically between normal tissue and the advancing tumor which is termed *shelving.* The proximal esophagus usually demonstrates very little dilatation.

Diverticula (Fig. 8-7). Esophageal diverticula are relatively common. Traction diverticula occur secondary to scarring from an adjacent disease process, e.g., tuberculosis, and are triangular in shape with the apex of the triangle pulled toward the diseased area. Traction diverticula occur more frequently in the middle third of the esophagus. Pulsion diverticula result from a weakness in the wall of the esophagus and are seen as rounded projections with a narrow neck. These are found more commonly in the upper and lower thirds of the esophagus. A Zenker's diverticulum is a pulsion diverticulum of the upper esophagus. An epiphrenic diverticulum is, as the name indicates, a pulsion diverticulum located just above the hemidiaphragm. Diverticula usually give no symptoms until they have reached a large size. Then, particularly in the upper esophagus, they may collect such a volume of food and secretions that a mechanical obstruction results. Also, when the patient is recumbent, the diverticulum may drain and be aspirated into the bronchi, creating a chronically relapsing pneumonitis.

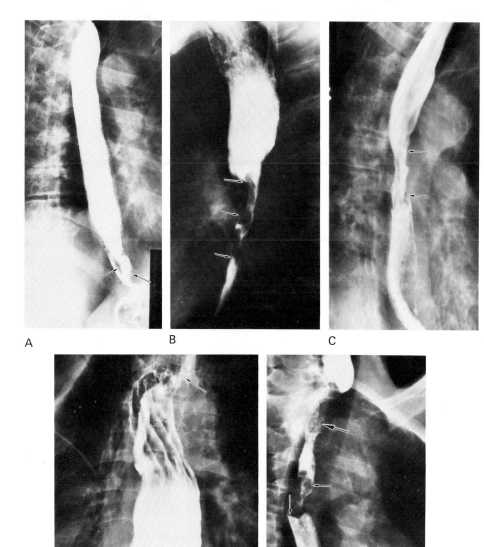

Fig. 8-5.

(A) Early adenocarcinoma of stomach, invading distal esophagus. The patient was biop-
sied on three occasions before the changes in the distal esophagus were confirmed. There
are only minor mucosal irregularities at the distal esophagus which could easily be overlooked.

(B) Large squamous cell carcinoma of distal esophagus. It is unusual to see the esophagus
this dilated proximal to carcinoma.

(C) Squamous cell carcinoma of midesophagus. (D) Same patient as (C) after esophagec-
tomy and esophagogastrostomy. The large arrow points to the cardiac silhouette and the
small arrow to the esophageal remnant.

(E) Large squamous cell carcinoma of the upper esophagus. Notice the abrupt change
between the normal mucosa and the tumor which produces "shelving," one of the hallmarks
of tumors of this type (small arrow). Also note the retained food particles in the upper
esophagus (large arrow).

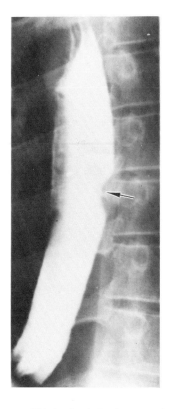

Fig. 8-6.
   Leiomyoma of midesophagus. This benign lesion has smooth margins and presents as a filling defect in the wall of the esophagus.

Varices (Fig. 8-8). These are varicose veins of the esophagus which arise due to an increased pressure within the portal venous system. When the pressure within the portal system increases above a certain level due to resistance to flow through the liver, the gastric and esophageal veins form a bypass to the systemic venous drainage and thus enlarge due to the increased blood flow. Demonstrable esophageal varices are usually associated with an enlarged spleen.

   Symptoms referable to varices include mild dysphagia and hematemesis. Melena may occur suddenly. Bleeding may be sufficient to cause cardiovascular shock. An antecedent history of liver cirrhosis is usually obtainable.

   One must be aware of the possibility of esophageal varices. Normally, when the esophagus is examined, the lumen is distended with barium to reveal subtle lesions; and this pressure may obliterate roentgen signs of varices. If the lumen of the esophagus is coated rather than distended with barium, varices appear as wormlike defects in the barium column. It is also worthy of note that varices

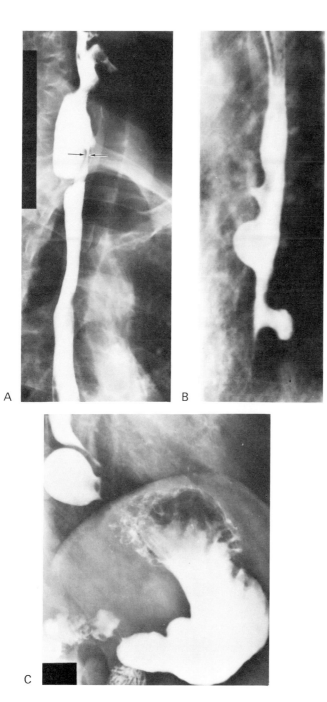

Fig. 8-7.
   Diverticula of the esophagus. (A) Zenker's (pulsion) diverticulum. This diverticulum is wider than the esophagus. The esophagus is narrow where it joins the diverticulum (arrows). (B) Traction diverticula secondary to tuberculosis. Notice the wide base and triangular shape. (C) Epiphrenic (pulsion) diverticulum. Notice how the diverticulum compresses the distal esophagus.

141

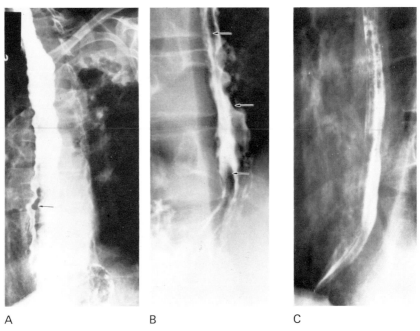

A   B   C

Fig. 8-8.

   (A) Large varices producing wormlike defects in the barium column. (B) Large varices seen on barium-coated esophageal film. (C) Same as (B) following a Warren shunt, which is a surgical procedure designed to shunt portal blood to the systemic system. This is a remark-able decrease in the size of the varices.

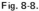

may not be demonstrated in the upright position but become readily apparent when the patient is recumbent. Physiologically, this occurs due to a decreased filling of the varices, with pooling of blood in the splanchnic bed when the patient is upright and a shift of the blood pool when the patient is recumbent.

Hiatal Hernia. By convention, hiatal hernia (Fig. 8-9) is a condition in which abdominal viscera herniate through a defect in the hemidiaphragm. The exact pathogenesis of hiatal hernia is not well understood, but generally there is a degradation, either congenital or acquired, of the phrenoesophageal membrane which firmly anchors the distal esophagus in its proper position.

   Hiatal hernias are common occurrences, being seen in approximately half the population. The percentage of occurrence goes up or down depending upon what criteria are used to make the diagnosis and to what extent the examiner pursues the demonstration. For example, if a patient is placed in the RAO position on the fluoroscope table and performs the Valsalva maneuver, a hiatal hernia will be demonstrated in 50 to 60 percent of the cases. If this maneuver is not used, perhaps only 20 percent of the patients will show a hiatal hernia.

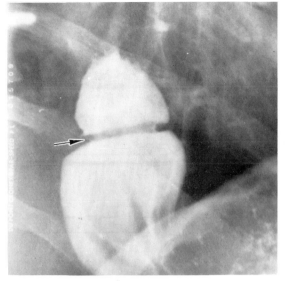

A

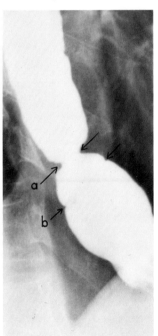

B

Figure 8-9.
(Legend on page 145.)

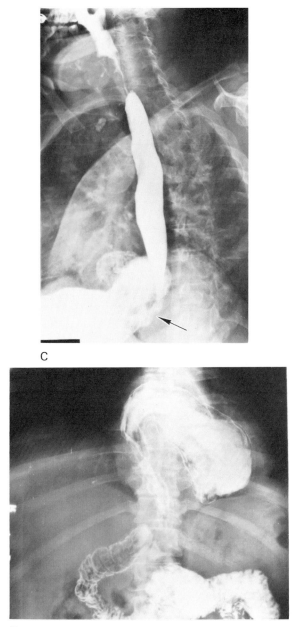

C

D

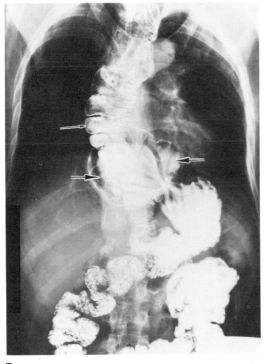

E

Fig. 8-9.

(A) Schatzki ring type hiatal hernia. (B) Esophageal peristaltic wave (a) (contraction ring) above a wide Schatzki ring (b). (C) Paraesophageal hernia. Notice the distal esophagus (arrow) is in its normal anatomical location. (D) Intrathoracic stomach. The entire stomach is in the thorax. (E) Colon bypass swing with large sliding hiatal hernia. Compare the appearance of the colonic (small arrow) to the gastric mucosa (large arrow).

Symptoms of hiatal hernia include heartburn, dysphagia, and pain. Most of these symptoms are related to reflux esophagitis. The examiner should be aware that pain from hiatal hernia may mimic coronary pain with the same pain distribution, and vice versa. If the hernia is large enough, compression of the mediastinal structures will result in an exaggerated substernal fullness and perhaps shortness of breath. A hiatal hernia is significant only if it relates to the patient's symptoms; otherwise, it should be noted only as an incidental finding.

Two types of hiatal hernia are seen roentgenographically. The sliding hernia is noted when a portion of the stomach slides above the hemidiaphragm, through the normal hiatus. Positive roentgenographic criteria for the presence of a sliding hernia have been the subject of controversy. The presence of a small portion of gastric mucosa above the level of the hemidiaphragm is thought to be meaningless, since the distal esophagus may contain such mucosa. The only acceptable, reliable sign of this type of hiatal hernia is the presence of a Schatzki ring, which is considered by most authorities to represent the junction between the esophagus and the stomach. A Schatzki ring is thought to develop as a defense mechanism against gastric reflux. The caliber of the ring may measure from 10 to 30 mm. If the diameter of the ring is less than 12 mm, and particularly if the patient has poor mastication, symptoms of dysphagia may be present. If the ring is greater than 28 mm, it is termed a *web* and probably has no clinical significance. On occasion, an obvious hiatal hernia with a large portion of the stomach above the hemidiaphragm may be noted without a Schatzki ring being present. On some occasions the entire stomach may slip through the hiatus, producing what is termed an *intrathoracic stomach*. Such hernias are usually associated with a congenitally shortened esophagus.

The other type of hernia occurs when the stomach or other viscera herniate through an opening adjacent to the esophageal hiatus. Since in this type of condition the distal esophagus remains in its normal location, the cardiac sphincter may be intact and the only symptom the patient may have is fullness in the chest, particularly after meals. Peptic erosion of the herniated stomach may also arise, creating symptoms referable to peptic or gastric ulcer.

Gastric Reflux. As with hiatal hernia, gastric reflux may be easily demonstrated. If reflux is persistent, erosion of the protective mucosa of the distal esophagus may occur and produce heartburn and pain. The severity of symptoms ranges from none at all to severe chest pain. The amount of protective mucus lining the esophagus and the acidity of the gastric contents also affect the severity and duration of symptoms referable to gastric reflux or heartburn. Reflux occurs more freely when the patient is straining or stooping. Anything which produces an increase in abdominal pressure can produce reflux in otherwise asymptomatic patients. Reflux may occur in association with hiatal hernia or without it. Reflux is the rule, rather than the exception, in pregnant women, particularly during the third trimester.

STOMACH, DUODENUM, AND SMALL BOWEL

The distal esophagus opens directly into the stomach through the cardiac orifice. Sizes and shapes of the stomach are so varied that almost any combination is considered to be normal. Through experience, one may determine a stomach to be "small" or "large"; but there really is no profile to use in evaluating gastric size and shape. The stomach (Fig. 8-10) occupies the medial portion of the left upper quadrant, with the cardiac orifice generally at the level of T-10 or T-11

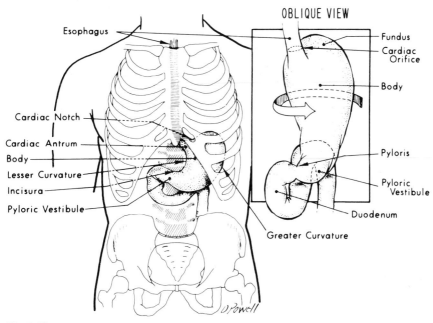

Fig. 8-10.
Anatomical relationships of stomach, duodenal bulb, and loop.

and the distal orifice (pyloric canal) located just to the right of L-1 or L-2. The "cap" portion of the stomach about the cardiac orifice is called the *fundus.* The major portion of the stomach extending from the fundus to a normal-appearing indenture (incisura) of the stomach wall is called the *body* of the stomach. The remaining portion of the distal stomach is called the *pyloric antrum* or, more commonly, *antrum.* The upper border of the stomach extending from the cardiac orifice to the antrum is termed the *lesser curvature,* and the lower border of the stomach in the same area is called the *greater curvature.* These curvatures show as smooth contours, and seldom are mucosal folds seen along the lesser curvature as compared to the common appearance of mucosal serrations along the greater curvature. Figure 8-11 illustrates a normal roentgenographic examination.

Appreciable peristalsis begins in the upper portion of the body of the stomach and gradually increases in intensity as it progresses toward the pyloric canal. As pressure in the antrum increases above the pressure in the duodenal bulb, the pyloric canal opens to allow the gastric contents to flow into the duodenal lumen. In the presence of inflammatory or mass lesions, peristalsis may be delayed or absent in that particular area; and in such a case, peristalsis becomes pathological.

The duodenal bulb is located adjacent to the pyloric channel. The appearance

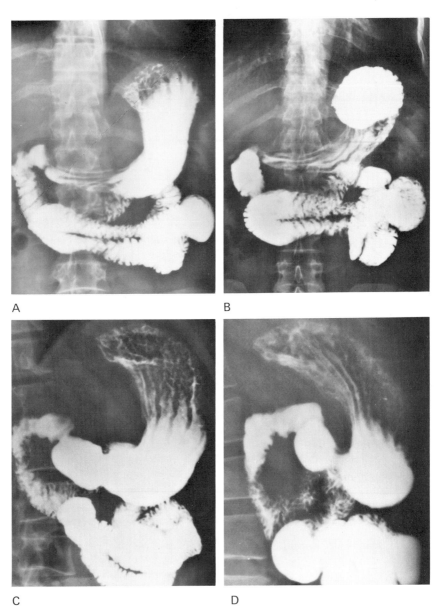

A

B

C

D

Fig. 8-11.

Normal upper gastrointestinal series. Compare to Figure 8-9. (A) Posteroanterior; (B) anteroposterior; (C) right anterior oblique; and (D) lateral views. Notice how the barium fills the fundus of the stomach on the AP view and the body on the PA view.

of the bulb has been described as that of a Christmas tree, with the trunk being the pyloric channel. The duodenal loop appears as a smooth C shape, with the tail of the C ending at the ligament of Treitz and the jejunum beginning at the termination of the duodenum. The jejunum is approximately eight feet long and coils in the left upper quadrant. It forms a loop in the opposite upper quadrant before terminating in the ileum. The ileum coils through the lower quadrants before terminating at the ileocecal valve on the inner aspect of the cecum of the colon.

The mucosa of the stomach appears as longitudinal ridges beginning at the upper portion of the stomach and radiating toward the pyloric canal. The mucosa of the duodenum appears as transverse ridges. In contrast, jejunal mucosa appears roentgenographically as small flecks of barium retained in mucosal folds corresponding to the outline of the bowel. Ileal folds are similar to duodenal folds but are not as broad and appear roentgenographically as transverse ridges in the barium column. Knowledge of mucosal appearance is important in localizing areas of bowel obstruction, particularly since entrapped bowel air may illustrate the mucosa (Fig. 8-12).

The anatomical position of the stomach and duodenum is of particular importance in evaluating abdominal pathology. The fundus of the stomach is in close proximity to the left hemidiaphragm superiorly and to the tail of the pancreas and spleen laterally and inferiorly. Normally the fundus of the stomach is within a half-centimeter of the left hemidiaphragm as seen in the recumbent view. If this distance is increased, one may suspect a space-occupying lesion between the stomach and the hemidiaphragm. One should correlate this finding with a lateral film of the stomach, since occasionally the apparently displaced stomach may be a matter of x-ray projection rather than true pathology. The posterior body of the stomach is adjacent to the body of the pancreas, the aorta, and the periaortic lymph nodes. The antrum, duodenal bulb, and loop are adjacent to the biliary system and to the head of the pancreas. Knowledge of the anatomical location of these organs may allow one to examine the stomach roentgenographically when looking for secondary evidence of a disease process elsewhere.

Complaints arising from the gastrointestinal tract may be nonspecific, and a meticulous medical history must be obtained from the patient to guide the radiologist in the search for pathology. One must also understand that the gastrointestinal tract may reflect psychological and emotional disturbances, as evidenced by the so-called gripping students may have in the abdominal area prior to examinations and to the increased occurrence of peptic ulcer disease in the spring and fall of the year.

Roentgenographic Examinations. Radiologists perform the majority of examinations of the stomach using barium sulfate to outline the inner walls of the gastrointestinal tract. The main purposes of examining the stomach or gastrointestinal tract are:

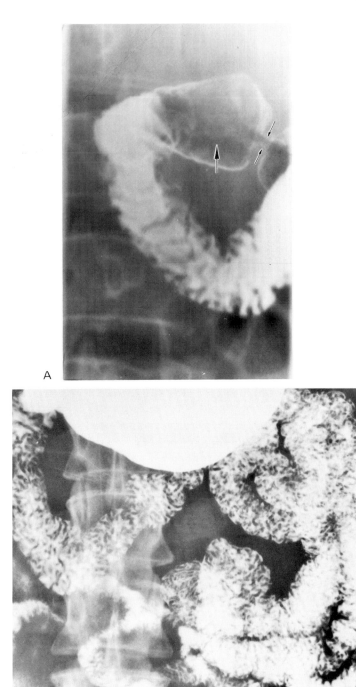

A

B

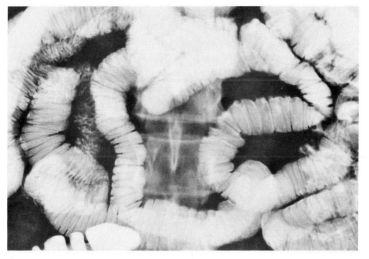

C

Fig. 8-12.

(A) A normal air-contrast study of the pyloric canal (small arrow), duodenal bulb (large arrow), and loop. (B) Normal jejunal mucosa. (C) Normal ileal mucosa.

1. To confirm peptic ulcer disease and follow the progress of treatment
2. To establish a diagnosis or suspicion of malignancy
3. To establish an etiology of acute or occult blood loss
4. To establish anatomical and physiological patterns, and
5. To locate masses outside the gastrointestinal tract

One should also mention several nonroentgenographic examinations which are routinely used in examination of the gastrointestinal tract and particularly the stomach. One of the most common is histamine stimulation of the stomach to produce acid. As a general statement, the presence of free acid excludes Addison's disease, pernicious anemia, and possibly gastric carcinoma, since it has been shown that antacidity may be present in these disease states. Demonstration of marked hyperacidity may also be used as an indication of how successfully one may expect to treat peptic ulcer disease. With the introduction of the gastric fibroscopes and cameras, a new dimension has been added to roentgenographic examinations, providing at least the possibility of examining a suspicious area seen at fluoroscopy. Unless one falls into the ever-present trap, positive information from gastroscopy is diagnostic if interpreted correctly; and negative information is not conclusive if pathological changes have been demonstrated roentgenographically. In our experience, gastric cytology has not been very beneficial in the diagnosis of gastrointestinal malignancies.

One further word should be stated concerning the preparation of the patient for examination of the gastrointestinal tract. Obviously, there is no preparation needed for examination of the esophagus, as it normally does not contain fluid or food particles. The standard preparation for an upper gastrointestinal series is for the patient to have nothing by mouth for at least six hours prior to examination of the stomach. Occasionally a patient may have a glass of water or other fluid several hours before the examination without presenting any problem. The rate of gastric emptying varies from patient to patient, but generally after a six-hour fast the stomach will be empty of all fluid and food particles. Occasionally, however, a patient will produce an excessive amount of fluid secretions in the stomach so that small amounts may always be present. In examination of the small bowel, care should be taken that there is no residual barium from a previous examination present to obscure pathology in the small bowel; as much cleansing of the small bowel as possible should be obtained. The greatest problem in preparation of the patient is eliminating all the feces from the colon which, in some institutions, appears almost impossible. A number of preparations are available to help rid the colon of feces; but overall, probably the best preparation is to put the patient on a low-residue or liquid diet and cathartics for a period of three days before the examination of the colon and to have a cleansing enema the morning of the examination. If even small particles of feces are present, the radiologist may have difficulty determining whether these are really fecal particles or whether they represent colonic polyps.

The preceding discussion presents the information we believe the student should know. Obviously great attention to detail must be given in examining the stomach to prevent subtle changes from being overlooked. In the next few paragraphs, we shall look at some of the common disease entities which relate to the stomach and correlate some basic medical information with roentgenographic findings.

Peptic and Duodenal Ulcers. By definition, a peptic ulcer is a crater produced by acid digestion and necrosis of the bowel wall. An ulcer is distinguished from an erosion in that an erosion involves the mucosa only, whereas an ulcer actually penetrates into the muscle layers of the bowel. Erosions are not generally seen roentgenographically. Ulcers most commonly occur in the distal esophagus, stomach, duodenum, and occasionally in the upper small bowel. Peptic ulceration is much more common in the duodenal bulb than in the stomach. Men are more commonly affected than women, and the typical age is mid-thirties for duodenal ulcers and mid-forties for gastric ulcers.

A chief symptom referable to peptic ulcer disease is pain, usually located in the epigastrium and occasionally radiating to other parts of the abdomen. Epigastric pain radiating to the back may indicate perforation into the pancreas. Pain from peptic ulcer disease is quite typical, and its hallmark is its relationship to food or antacid intake. The cyclic gnawing or burning pain will be relieved by

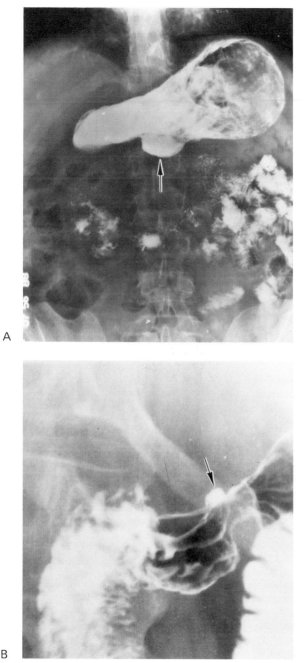

A

B

Figure 8-13.
(Legend on page 155.)

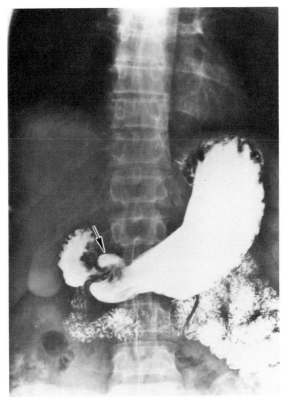

C

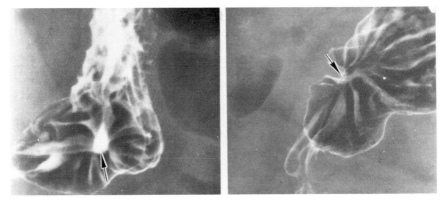

D

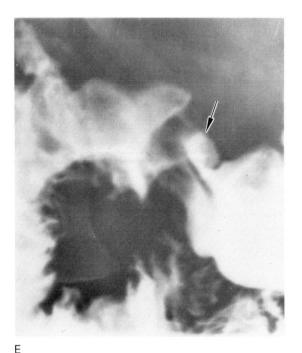

E

Fig. 8-13.

Benign gastric ulcers. (A) Large benign greater curvature ulcer with retained gastric secretions and food particles. (B) Lesser curvature ulcer shown on air-contrast study. (C) Penetrating prepyloric lesser curvature ulcer. (D) Two views of posterior ulcer with resultant scarring. (E) Pyloric channel ulcer. It is very difficult at times to ascertain the exact anatomical location of an ulcer. On occasion the radiologist will refer to *juxtapyloric* to indicate that an ulcer is in the vicinity of the pyloric canal.

food ingestion; relief will last until the stomach is emptied, with pain then recurring. Pain from peptic ulceration of the pyloric channel may be accentuated by food intake due to increased gastric peristalsis with resultant increased pressure against the diseased area. Occasionally pain from gastric ulcers may be accentuated by meals and relieved by antacid, since food may stimulate peristalsis and irritate the ulcer. Weight loss and diarrhea are uncommon in peptic ulcer disease unless the disease is complicated by obstruction or fistula.

Roentgenographically, gastric ulcers (Fig. 8-13) appear as outpouchings from the stomach wall. Face on, the appearance is that of a crater with a radiating, spokelike wheel of mucosal folds running to the edge of the crater. The presence of radiating folds, penetration of the ulcer through the stomach wall, and evidence of complete healing are the only reliable signs one should depend upon in determining whether an ulcer is benign or not. The presence of a concomitant duodenal ulcer is also strong evidence for a benign gastric ulcer.

In contrast to benign ulcers, malignant ulcers may show roentgenographic evidence of an associated mass. Radiating folds may be present, but the folds terminate at the edge of the mass rather than at the brink of the ulcer crater. A particular location along the greater or lesser curvature of the stomach is not a reliable sign in differentiating one lesion in itself. Differentiation between benign and malignant conditions may be extremely difficult. Some malignant ulcers have also been noted to show some signs of healing and thus have been misinterpreted as benign ulcers.

Complications from gastric ulcers include obstruction, bleeding, and perforation and are also considered indications for surgery. As gastric ulcers heal, only a small residual scar remains; and normal peristalsis again proceeds through the scarred area. It is uncommon for gastric ulcers to produce scarring significant enough to deform the outline of the stomach.

Duodenal ulcers (Fig. 8-14) produce the same picture as gastric ulcers, although they are generally smaller. Edema and radiating folds may not be as prominent as they are in gastric ulcers, and the radiologist may have to resort to films taken while the duodenal bulb is being compressed to demonstrate the ulcer niche. Duodenal ulcers occur mostly in the bulb and are occasionally seen in the second portion of the duodenal loop. In contrast to gastric ulcers, ulcers of the duodenum may scar, producing obstruction or a typical deformity of the bulb. In the presence of scarring, it may be difficult to differentiate active ulcers from chronic scarring. A roentgenographic report depicting a scarred duodenal bulb indicates that the patient has had peptic ulcer disease, and no inference can be made concerning its activity. If the patient is asymptomatic, one may conclude that no active disease is present. If he is symptomatic, the presence of active disease is implied.

Particular severity and atypical location of peptic ulcers occurs in Zollinger-Ellison syndrome, which is a disease process due to increased acid production from gastric glands secondary to a gastrin-producing tumor that is usually located in the pancreas.

Reexamination of patients with ulcer disease is, simply stated, overdone. Reexamination of an asymptomatic patient with previous demonstrated duodenal ulcer is generally not indicated. In contrast, reexamination of gastric ulcer patients following a course of medical management is indicated, since there are occasions in which a benign-appearing ulcer in the stomach may actually be malignant. (Most gastroenterologists believe that good management of a gastric ulcer can be achieved only with the patient in the hospital!) On some occasions the radiologist may request a repeat examination of an area suspicious for an active ulcer to reconfirm or disavow his suspicions.

Gastritis. Although peptic ulcer disease is one of the most common reasons for examining the stomach and duodenum, other entities are also commonly seen.

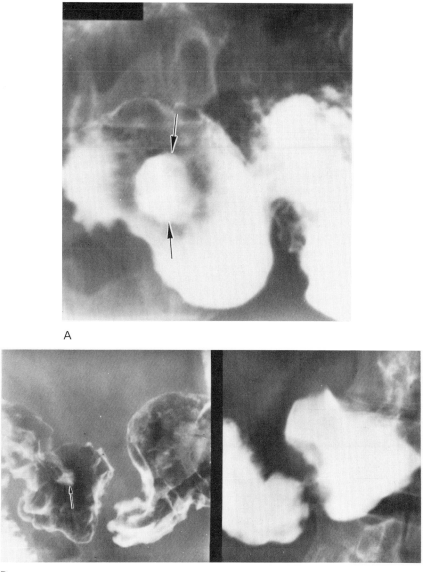

A

B

Figure 8-14.
(Legend on page 159.)

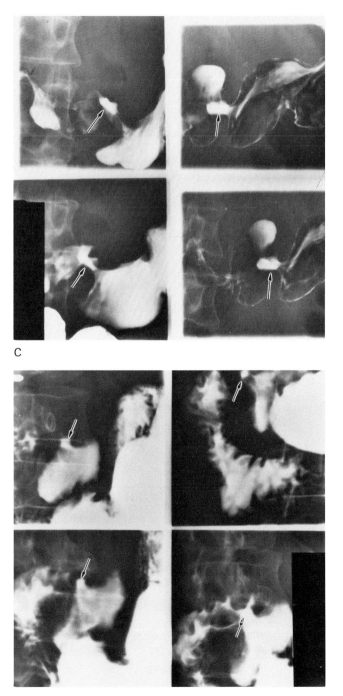

C

D

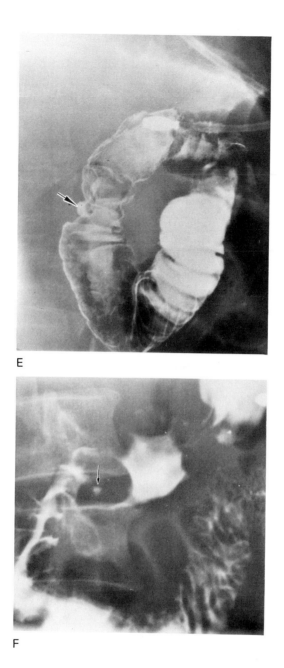

E

F

Fig. 8-14.

    Duodenal ulcers. (A) Active duodenal ulcer of bulb. (B) Active duodenal ulcer (arrow) shown on air-contrast examination but not seen on the prone film. The barium filled and air-contrast views are variants of the standard of obtaining two views of each area of interest. (C) Healed pyloric channel ulcer presenting as a pseudodiverticulum with both barium and air contrast views. (D) Active ulcer in distal bulb. (E) Postbulbar ulcer shown on hypotonic duodenography. (F) Aberrant pancreas in duodenal bulb. Note the resemblance to an active ulcer. The arrow points to the duct entering the aberrant pancreas.

Vague abdominal pain with no particular etiology suspected is a common clinical symptom necessitating examination of the upper gastrointestinal tract. Gastritis, either from a viral or alcoholic etiology, may produce superficial changes in the gastric mucosa which can be readily seen with the gastroscope but with no changes noted roentgenographically. Although alcohol is a depressant rather than a stimulant, it does increase acid and mucus production in the stomach. The result is that the gastric mucosa becomes congested and hyperemic and easily bleeds. The patient with alcoholic gastritis may present with severe blood loss with no changes shown on the upper gastrointestinal series.

Atrophic gastritis as seen in pernicious anemia appears to be a common clinical condition which is difficult to demonstrate roentgenographically. In patients with pernicious anemia, loss of the gastric rugae with the resultant smoothing of the greater curvature of the stomach suggests gastric atrophy; but this occurs in less than half the patients with pernicious anemia.

Tumors. Among stomach lesions, tumors are quite common. The vast majority are adenocarcinomas of one type or another, with only a small number of these tumors being sarcomas such as a reticulum cell sarcoma, lymphosarcoma, Hodgkin's disease, or leiomyosarcoma. Symptoms of gastric tumors are vague in nature and often present as bleeding or outlet obstruction. Loss of appetite, weight loss, and early satiety also suggest the presence of a gastric tumor.

Roentgenographically, gastric tumors (Fig. 8-15) present as filling defects in the gastric wall, with abnormal peristalsis seen fluoroscopically. Some degree of rigidity is usually also present. The filling defects may present as an ulcerating mass with ragged mucosa, as polypoid defects, or possibly as infiltration of the mucosa and muscular layers of the stomach associated with fixation of the stomach. Tumors in the antrum tend to obstruct the pyloric canal; whereas lesions of the cardia may invade the esophagus and the patient may present with symptoms of dysphagia. Complications of gastric tumors are the same as for benign gastric ulcers. Differentiating between sarcoma and carcinoma may be difficult roentgenographically. Sarcoma tends to have a more polypoid appearance than carcinoma, but this is not always true (Fig. 8-16). Infiltrating tumors such as carcinoma may present roentgenographically with prominent mucosal folds such as might be seen in hypertrophic gastritis or Menetrier's disease.

Benign tumors of the stomach are usually adenomatous polyps or leiomyomata. These appear as a single polypoid or a multiple polypoid-appearing mass. Generally there is no fixation of the stomach wall, and peristalsis may proceed normally.

Prolapse of Gastric Mucosa. Prolapse into the base of the duodenal bulb is a common finding. This prolapse occurs because of loose attachment of the mucosa to the gastric musculature and hyperperistalsis or strong peristalsis

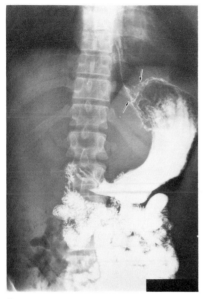

A

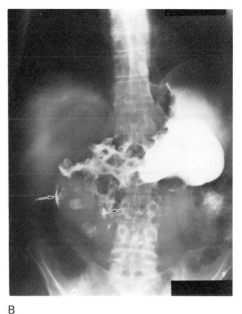

B

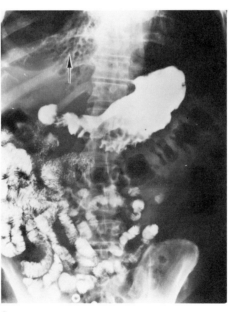

C

Fig. 8-15.

Gastric carcinomas. (A) Adenocarcinoma of stomach, invading esophagus. (B) Huge adenocarcinoma of stomach with perforation. Arrows outline barium within the peritoneal cavity. (C) Adenocarcinoma of greater curvature. Notice the bronchiectasis of the right lower lung.

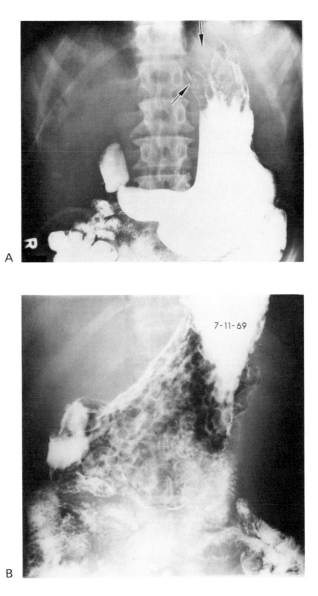

Fig. 8-16.
   Gastric sarcomas. (A) Hodgkin's disease. Although more prominent, the mucosal changes are similar to those seen in Figure 8-15A. (B) Lymphosarcoma of the stomach. This patient survived seven years with this tumor.

pushing the mucosa through the pyloric channel. Prolapse has little clinical significance, although there have been recent reports that there may be occult
bleeding at its site.

Gastric Anastomoses. Before leaving the subject of the stomach, a few words
should be stated concerning operative anastomoses (Fig. 8-17). A gastroenterostomy is a drainage procedure in which a loop of small bowel (usually duodenum or upper jejunum) is anastomosed to the inferior aspect of the stomach.
Antrectomy is resection of the antrum with anastomosis between the gastric
remnant and the pyloric canal. Pyloroplasty is incision and oversewing of the
pyloric canal. Vagotomy is resection and interruption of the vagus nerves to
decrease acid production in the stomach. A Billroth I gastroenterostomy is a
partial gastrectomy with anastomosis between the gastric remnants and the
duodenum. A Billroth II gastroenterostomy is a partial gastrectomy with
anastomosis between the gastric remnants and the jejunum.

Pancreatic Disease. Perhaps one of the more challenging examinations of the
upper gastrointestinal tract is that of the duodenal loop for evidence of pancreatitis or pancreatic carcinoma. Pancreatitis is inflammation of the pancreas
caused either by alcoholism, gallstones, trauma, or viral infections. Onset of
symptoms is sudden, with severe midepigastric pain which may bore through to
the back. There is usually associated nausea, vomiting, and bloating due to
reflex ileus of the adjacent bowel.

Roentgenographically, only 20 to 25 percent of patients will demonstrate
signs of pancreatitis (Fig. 8-18). If present, roentgen signs may involve the
inferior aspect of the antrum and/or the inner aspects of the first, second, or
third portions of the duodenal loop. Edematous changes of the mucosa of the
upper loop are most commonly seen, and on occasion there is effacement of
the mucosa in the same area.

With acute attacks, sterile abscesses (pseudocysts) may develop which slowly
resolve (Fig. 8-19). On occasion, these pseudocysts persist and become quite
large, enlarging the duodenal loop and sometimes producing large lesions in
the middle or left upper abdominal region. Pseudocysts may be treated surgically by complete removal or marsupialization into the stomach or small bowel.

Insidious onset of painless jaundice is typical of tumor involving the head
of the pancreas. Roentgen signs of this tumor are generally the same as for
pancreatitis. Tumors involving the body or tail of the pancreas may efface
the stomach and produce symptoms referable to gastric ulcers (Fig. 8-20).

Small Bowel Disease. Diseases of the small bowel are not as commonly seen
roentgenographically as disease processes of the stomach and duodenum. Parasitic infestation, tumors, regional enteritis, and malabsorption syndromes are
the most common processes seen. Of these, regional enteritis appears to be
more common.

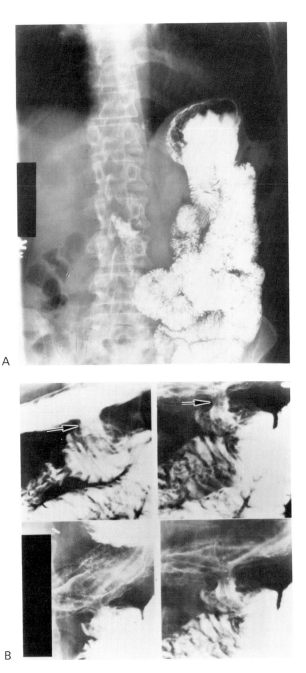

A

B

Fig. 8-17.
Postoperative appearance of anastomoses. (A) Billroth II gastroenterostomy. The gastric remnant empties directly into the jejunum without going into the duodenum. (B) Spot films of gastroenterostomy. This is a drainage procedure. The stomach is located above and the jejunum below.

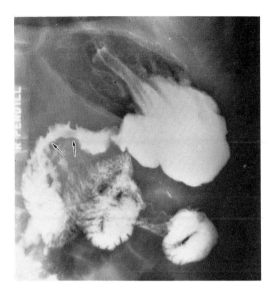

Fig. 8-18.
Pancreatitis. Notice the effacement of the inner aspects of the duodenal loop. These changes may also be seen in pancreatic carcinoma.

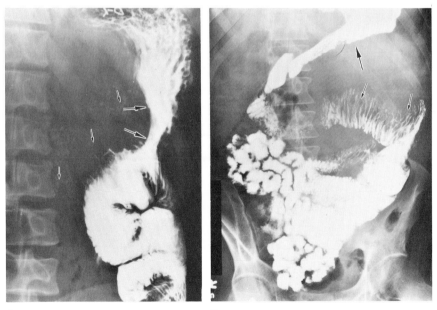

A   B

Fig. 8-19.
(A) Pancreatitis displacing the stomach anteriorly. Notice all the calcification in the pancreas. (B) Large pancreatic pseudocyst displacing the stomach and effacing the small bowel. The small bowel is dilated and edematous in proximity to the pseudocyst.

165

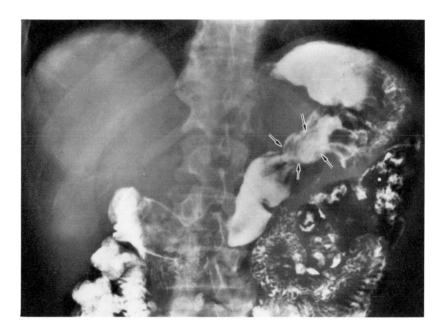

Fig. 8-20.
    Gastric ulcer secondary to invasion of the stomach by carcinoma of the pancreas. This is a good example of how one may use an upper gastrointestinal series to demonstrate disease in an adjacent organ.

Regional enteritis (Fig. 8-21) is of unknown etiology and occurs mostly in patients in the third or fourth decade of life. In acute cases, clinical symptoms may be suggestive of acute appendicitis or intestinal obstruction. It is primarily located in the terminal ileum but may be seen throughout the bowel. It may also present with mild intermittent diarrhea with abdominal cramps and possibly a bloody diarrhea. As the disease progresses, stenotic areas present clinically as partial bowel obstruction. Fistulas may also develop between loops of small bowel or other viscera. Roentgenographically, early disease may not be recognized; but as the disease progresses, the appearance of regional enteritis is that of edematous mucosa with spiking of the mucosa and local areas suggestive of small ulcerations. The terminal ileum should be visualized in all examinations, preferably by barium enema. If the barium cannot be refluxed through the ileocecal valve, a small bowel series should also be performed for complete evaluation of the small bowel mucosa.

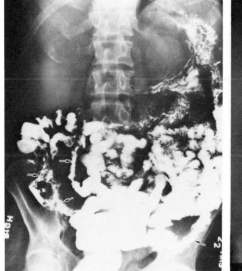 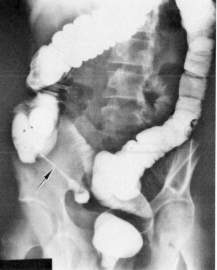

A   B

Fig. 8-21.
Regional enteritis. (A) Several areas of involvement are marked. The ileal folds are edematous and scarred. Ileal loops are separated, whereas normally they are within a few millimeters from one another. Compare to Figure 8-12C. (B) Long stricture of terminal ileum with dilated small bowel proximal to the stricture. Some patients have multiple strictures in the small bowel similar to this.

Diverticula (Fig. 8-22) of the bowel occur with great frequency. It is common to see duodenal diverticula arising from the medial border of the second and sometimes third portion of the duodenal loop. Diverticula are also seen in the small bowel, with more seen in the upper than the lower portion. Diverticula of the duodenum and small bowel usually have little significance, although on occasion they may become inflamed and perforate. Diverticula of the stomach are uncommon.

Tumors of the small bowel are infrequent. Most commonly they include such entities as lymphosarcoma and Hodgkin's disease.

In some of the recent medical literature there has been a great deal of comment concerning malabsorption syndromes involving the small bowel. Generally these malabsorption syndromes produce roentgenographic changes consistent with segmentation, i.e., separation of the barium column into fragments several centimeters in length; flocculation, i.e., clumping of the barium; and edematous changes within the mucosa. The References offer more specific details.

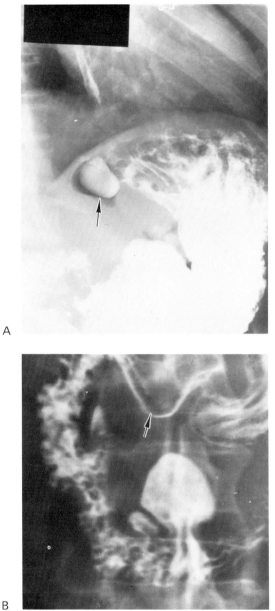

A

B

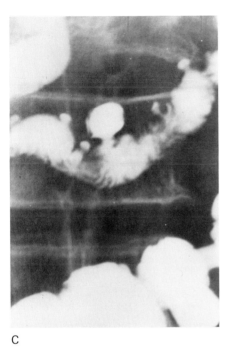 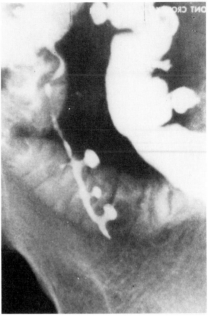

C   D

Fig. 8-22.
Diverticula. (A) Gastric diverticulum adjacent to the esophagogastric junction. (B) Duo-denal diverticula. The arrow points to the duodenal bulb. Three diverticula are seen. (C) Small bowel diverticula. (D) Diverticula of appendix. Small bowel diverticula are also noted. Some authorities believe that a patient should have an elective appendectomy for appendiceal diverticula since they so frequently rupture.

COLON

The large bowel extends from the terminal ileum to the anus. It is approximately six feet long and forms a modified arch beginning in the right lower quadrant and extending up to the liver and then across the epigastric region to the region of the spleen and then down through the left lower quadrant to the midline region of the pelvis. Several distinct regions are noted (Fig. 8-23). The cecum is the first portion of the colon and contains the orifices of the terminal ileum and appendix. The right or ascending colon, the hepatic flexure, transverse colon, splenic flexure, descending colon or left colon, sigmoid, rectum, and anus are the significant areas of the colon.

The appendix is a narrow tube usually arising from the inferior or medial aspect of the cecum and varies from 2 to 20 cm in length, averaging 8 to 10 cm long. The cecum is usually anterior, lying against the anterior abdominal wall

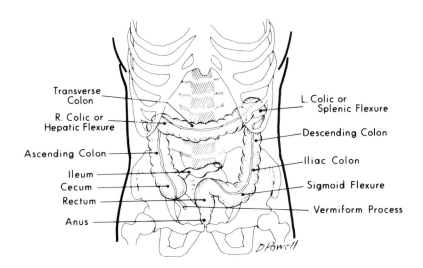

Fig. 8-23.
Anatomy of the colon.

and occasionally in the pelvis. As the colon ascends, it becomes more posterior
until it lies adjacent to the undersurface of the liver. The transverse colon is in
apposition with the greater curvature of the stomach and portions of the body
of the pancreas. As the transverse colon turns downward it is in contact with
the inferior surface of the spleen and forms the region of the splenic flexure
before becoming the left, or descending, colon. The sigmoid colon generally
lies within the pelvis and is usually extremely mobile. The distal portion of the
sigmoid colon is important in its relationships because behind it are the iliac
vessels and sacral nerves and in front are the bladder in the male and the uterus
in the female.

The sigmoid ends at the rectum, which is at the level of the third sacral ver-
tebra, and generally follows the curvature of the sacrum and coccyx to the
region of the anus. The distal part of the rectum dilates to form the rectal
ampulla and contains prominent transverse folds known as Houston's valves.
The rectum usually can be examined very easily with a sigmoidoscope and
because of overlying areas is not adequately examined roentgenographically.
The anus composes only the terminal one to two inches of the colon and has
no peritoneal covering, being invested by muscle groups.

Roentgenographic examination of the colon is performed by instilling barium
in such a fashion as to completely fill the lumen of the bowel and to obtain a
small amount of reflux through the terminal ileum (Fig. 8-24). Either the
terminal ileum, ileocecal valve, or appendix must be identified before it can

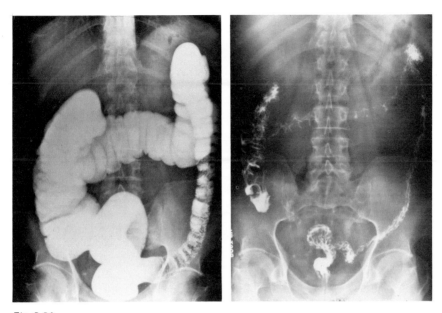

Fig. 8-24.
Normal barium enema (left) with evacuation film (right).

be absolutely certain that the cecum has been filled. There are occasions when the cecum is doubled under the right colon, and one may mistakenly fill only a portion of the colon and miss a carcinoma hiding in the cecum. The most important portion of the barium enema is the postevacuation film, in which the mucosal detail is fairly well outlined.

On occasion, an air-contrast barium examination of the colon may be performed to detect small lesions, particularly polypoid lesions (Fig. 8-25). The air-contrast examination is performed by first filling the colon with barium and then having the patient evacuate, and then partially filling the colon again with a thick barium mixture. Air is then pumped into the colon to produce a double-density air-contrast examination of the lumen of the bowel. The presence of even small particles of feces may create difficulty in differentiating fecal particles from polyps and sometimes small carcinomatous lesions of the colon.

Although there are numerous varieties of lesions involving the colon, only the more common ones to see in an average practice will be discussed. Congenital lesions such as imperforate anus, malrotation, and colonic atresia are adequately covered in other textbooks.

Diverticulosis (Fig. 8-26). There are two types of colonic diverticula, namely, congenital and acquired. Diverticula generally occur through weak places in the

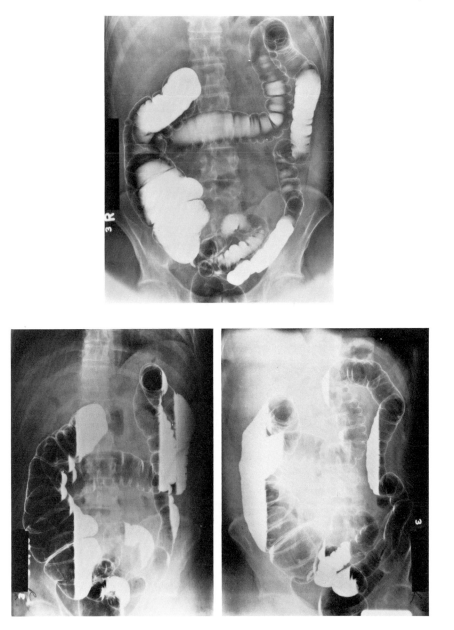

Fig. 8-25.

Normal air-contrast barium enema, AP and both decubitus films. The wall of the colon is more clearly demonstrated than in Figure 8-24.

muscular coat of the colon along the sites of insertion of the terminal branches of the mesenteric vessels into the bowel wall. Diverticula are most frequently seen along the sigmoid colon, but on occasion they may extend throughout the colon. The areas of diverticulosis may sometimes be associated with spasm, and thickened mucosal folds may be seen. Also the diverticula may become infected and perforate, producing periocolic abscesses. The diagnosis of diverticulitis (Fig. 8-27) in the presence of diverticulosis may be difficult and may depend upon the fluoroscopic examination of the radiologist. Clinically, diverticulosis may be asymptomatic or it may produce symptoms referable to low-grade infection and low-grade obstruction. Clinical signs may range from a slight soreness in the left lower quadrant to the symptoms of peritonitis and perforation. Diverticulosis is more common after the age of 50 and apparently increases with the age of the patient.

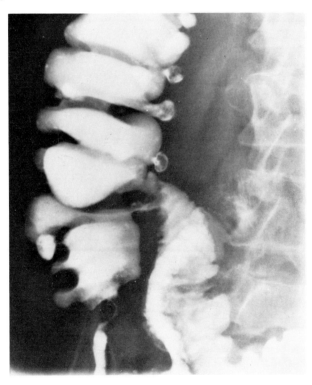

Fig. 8-26.
  Diverticulosis of right colon. Diverticula are more commonly seen in the sigmoid colon.

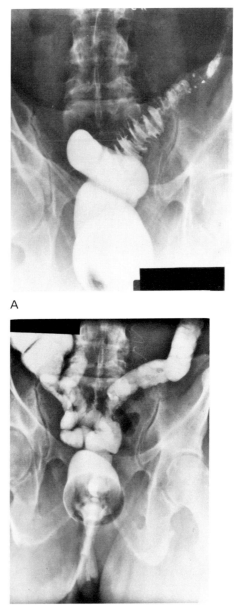

A

B

Fig. 8-27.

(A) Diverticulitis of sigmoid colon. The colonic mucosa is edematous and, as in this patient, numerous diverticula may not be seen. (B) Same patient postoperatively.

Colonic Polyps (Fig. 8-28). Two types of polyps are generally recognized roent-genographically, namely, the adenomatous type, which are sacular projections into the lumen of the bowel, and the villous polyps, which are broad-based and also project into the colonic lumen. Polyps are more frequently noted in the left colon than in the right. From chronic irritation, polyps may ulcerate and bleed, producing symptoms of an irritable bowel or diarrhea. Although there is a rather heated discussion among some physicians about colonic polyps, it is generally conceded that a single polyp measuring less than 2.5 cm may be watched roent-genographically. If any sign of enlargement is noted, the polyp should be removed. Any polyp suspected as the site of bleeding generally is removed. Familial polyps may occur throughout the entire small bowel and colon and may produce symptoms of widespread bleeding and irritation. They carry with them the high risk of malignant degeneration.

Carcinoma of the Colon (Fig. 8-29). Carcinoma of the colon generally is adeno-carcinoma, with the sarcomas not commonly seen. About 75 percent of colonic carcinomas occur in the rectosigmoid area, and it is generally believed that most of these cancers can be found with adequate sigmoidoscopic examination. Symptoms may be referable to the location of the lesion. As with polyps, lesions

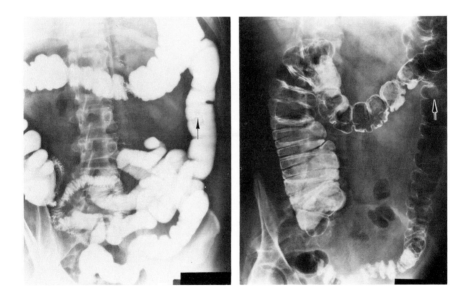

Fig. 8-28.
   Colonic polyp, left colon, with air-contrast examination. The narrow segment in the transverse colon is due to spasm.

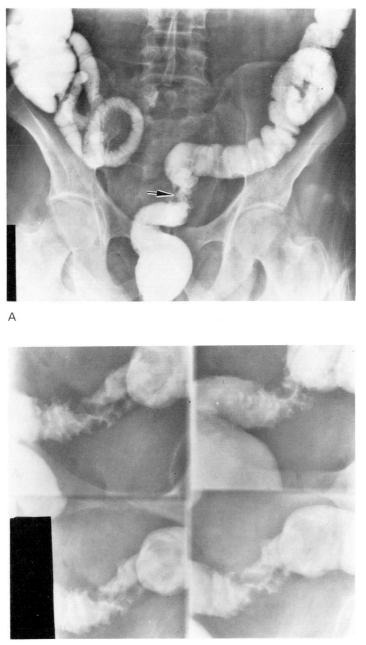

A

B

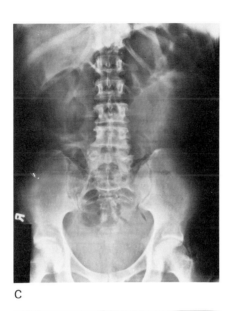

C

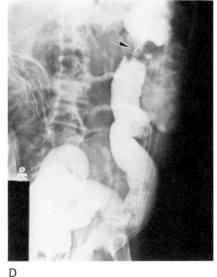

D

Fig. 8-29.
Carcinoma of the colon. (A, B) Adenocarcinoma of the sigmoid colon. Notice the mucosal destruction shown on the spot films.

(C, D) Adenocarcinoma of the left colon. The plain film shows increased air in the transverse colon. The barium enema shows a typical annular constriction of the colon that usually accompanies these tumors.

in the right colon may produce no early symptoms and may be found on routine evaluation for anemia, since these tumors may become quite large and ulcerate and bleed without producing significant symptoms. There is also more of a tendency for those in the right colon generally to penetrate the wall of the bowel and extend into the surrounding tissues rather than to encircle and obstruct the colon. Lesions in the left colon, where the diameter of the colon is smaller and the contents of the bowel less liquid, are more progressive, producing a napkin-ring type of growth and causing chronic obstructive symptoms and, occasionally, bleeding. Gross blood in the stools per se is more commonly seen in lesions of the left or sigmoid colon. Crampy abdominal pain may occur with tumors on either side but is generally infrequent with tumors involving the rectum. Perforation of the colon by malignant masses is generally not a presenting symptom and is more likely to occur with acute obstruction than with chronic obstruction. Volvulus and intussusception also occur but are unusual and generally secondary to a polypoid type of mass.

Roentgenographically, these tumors generally present as a filling defect in the barium-filled colon associated with mucosal destruction and change in the lumen of the bowel. It may be difficult on occasion to differentiate between a malignant process and an inflammatory lesion. Generally it is believed that carcinoma has a rather clear-cut transition from malignant mucosa to normal mucosa and that the length of involved bowel generally is shorter in carcinoma than in inflammatory lesions. The mucosa is actually destroyed by carcinomatous involvement; whereas inflammatory lesions on close inspection may show areas of normal bowel mucosa.

Colonic Obstruction and Irritation. Clinical symptoms referable to obstruction of the colon depend upon the nature of the lesion as well as the location. Bowel habits are important, and a change in these habits should lead one to examination of the colon. Examination of stools or material taken at sigmoidoscopy may reveal parasites, inflammatory cells, mucus, blood, or combinations of these. Laboratory examinations may show excessive amounts of fat, and biopsies taken may show mucosal changes in the bowel wall. Constipation is an objective symptom acknowledged by the patient and may mean many different things, such as a change in the number of stools, the time of day in which stools are passed, the character of the stools, or sensation of incomplete emptying of the rectum. These changes may be due to impairment of colonic mobility such as occurs in those who chronically take cathartics or they may be due to an actual obstructive lesion.

The irritable colon may produce no roentgenographic signs and is clinically highlighted by the presence of rhythmic, cramping pain and constipation, as are generally associated with the excessive use of cathartics. The so-called cathartic colon is commonly seen in elderly patients after they have taken large quantities of laxatives over a long period of time. The first roentgenographic changes are those of loss of the haustral markings and development of a smooth bowel wall. However, there is no rigidity or stiffening of the bowel wall, and there are no marked mucosal changes or true strictures as may be seen in ulcerative colitis.

Gastroenteritis, particularly secondary to bacterial or viral infection of the colon, occurs commonly. In the early examination there may be no roentgeno-graphic signs, although on occasion an atonic or irritable colon may be demon-strated. In chronic (spastic) colitis there may be spasm and loss of the normal mucosal pattern as seen also in the cathartic colon. Diverticuli are commonly

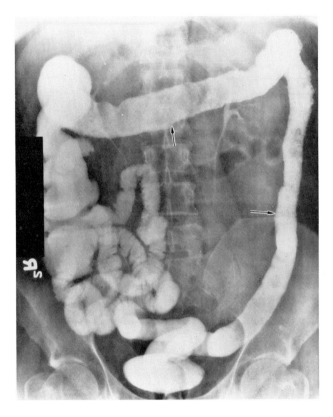

Fig. 8-30.
Ulcerative colitis, sparing rectosigmoid and right colon. The colitis extends from the region of the upper arrow to the lower arrow. Notice how irregular the mucosa is as compared to that in other areas. Contrast material is seen in the kidneys.

associated with the spastic colon. Parasitic infestations often show changes in
the cecum, roentgenographically demonstrated by a thickened wall of the
cecum associated with irregular mucosa and rarely with evidence of involvement
of the terminal ileum.

Ulcerative Colitis (Fig. 8-30). Ulcerative colitis usually occurs in young men
and presents clinically with excessive diarrhea and production of blood, pus,
and mucus in the stools. Ulcerative colitis should be contrasted with granulomatous colitis. Ulcerative colitis generally begins at the anus and ascends,
producing marked ulceration of mucosa. Granulomatous colitis (Fig. 8-31)
usually begins in the cecum and terminal ileum and descends and may have
lesions also involving other areas of the bowel. Following therapy, ulcerative
colitis may become quiescent, or it may become chronic and lead to long areas

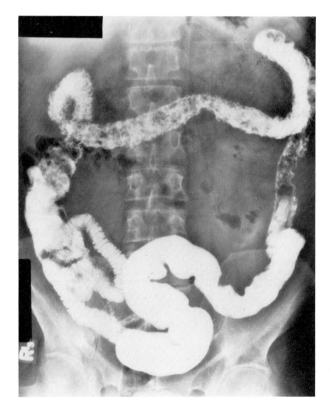

Fig. 8-31.
Granulomatous colitis extending from the cecum to the sigmoid colon.

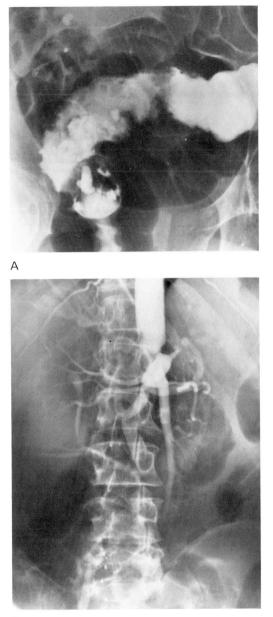

A

B

Fig. 8-32.

Ischemic rectosigmoiditis. (A) Barium enema. The colonic mucosa is abnormal from the sigmoid to the anus. (B) Aortogram demonstrating complete occlusion of the aorta, including the inferior mesenteric artery.

of stricture due to fibrosis in the healing of the ulcerative areas. Ulcerative colitis carries with it an increased frequency of carcinomatous changes, whereas granulomatous colitis apparently does not.

Vascular Insults (Fig. 8-32). Vascular insults to the colon may present as acute abdominal cramping pain. The typical clinical symptom is that of a patient having pain some two to three hours after ingestion of food. It is uncommon to have involvement of the colon without involvement of the small bowel. Partial occlusion of the mesenteric arterial supply may be without signs; but on occasion, bruits may be heard over the midback or abdomen. Roentgenographically one may see no change or one may see evidence of what are termed *pseudotumors* due to a collection of fluid or blood or both within the bowel walls producing what is known as a thumbprint sign. Vascular insults may affect the mobility of the colon, producing distention of the proximal unaffected portion with essentially a flat distal segment of bowel. Vascular insults may progress to areas of necrosis and perforation. Bowel infarction may also occur without evidence of occlusion of major vascular channels, as seen either at angiography or autopsy.

Intussusception is usually associated with the presence of a mass lesion within the bowel lumen. In adults this is most often secondary to polyps or carcinoma, and in the child it may be purely physiological. Volvulus is more commonly seen in adults and is usually secondary to the great mobility of the sigmoid colon and occasionally of the cecum. Due to the hypermobility and hypermotility of the colon, the sigmoid colon may wrap around itself, producing an acute obstructive lesion with all the secondary signs of obstruction. Roentgenographically one may see an abnormal amount of air within what would be the sigmoid colon, which should lead one to suspect the presence of a volvulus (see Chapter 6). Occasionally one may recognize a large amount of gas in what appears to be the cecum, located in the left upper quadrant, in which case a cecal volvulus should be suspected.

To reemphasize once more before concluding this chapter: before a barium enema can be completed, the patient must be given adequate bowel preparation. Cathartics should not be used in the preparation of patients with suspected obstruction, ulcerative colitis, or in the presence of active bleeding. In patients with loss of normal bowel habits, diarrhea, constipation, bleeding, or anemia, a barium enema may be requested as a portion of the patient's total evaluation.

READING LIST

Kyser, F. A., and McEwen, E. G. (Eds.). Diseases of the Digestive Tract. *Med. Clin. North Am.* vol. 48, no. 1, 1964.

Margolis, A. R., and Burhenne, H. J. *Alimentary Tract Roentgenology.* St. Louis: Mosby, 1967.

Marshak, R. H. (Ed.). Radiology of the Alimentary Tract. *Radiol. Clin. North Am.* vol. 7, no. 1, 1969.

Marshak, R. H., and Lindner, A. E. *Radiology of the Small Intestine.* Philadelphia: Saunders, 1970.

Michener, W. M. The Gastrointestinal Disorders. *Pediatr. Clin. North Am.* vol. 14, no. 1, 1967.

Zellman, H. E. (Ed.). Systemic Diseases in the Gastrointestinal Tract. *Med. Clin. North Am.* vol. 50, no. 2, 1966.

The Urinary Tract

9

THE KIDNEYS lie in the retroperitoneal fascial space, with the hilum of the right kidney at the level of L-2 and the hilum of the left at the level of L-1. The right kidney is slightly lower due to the presence of the adjacent liver. The lower poles of the kidneys are projected slightly laterally as they lie against the psoas muscles, producing a slight obliquity to the kidney axes. Each kidney measures roughly 10 to 12 cm in length and 4 to 5 cm in breadth. The kidneys weigh between 140 and 150 gm each and are generally larger in the male than in the female (Fig. 9-1).

The kidney is composed of an outer rim of cortex interposed between pyramids of medullary tissue. From the cortex arise the renal tubules consisting of glomeruli and associated blood vessels. Nephrons leading from the glomerular capsule course through the cortical and medullary substance, eventually emptying through the renal pyramids into the urinary collecting system. Surrounding each renal pyramid is a collecting tube, termed a *minor calyx.* Each calyx is shaped like a buttercup, and there is one minor calyx corresponding to each renal pyramid. The minor calyxes form four to five major calyxes, and these in turn form the renal pelvis (Fig. 9-2). Surrounding the kidneys is a layer of adipose tissue which, because of the density difference between fat and the soft tissue of the kidney, allows visualization of the renal shadows on the roentgenogram.

The relationship of the kidneys to other organs within the body is extremely important. Superior and slightly medial to the kidneys are the adrenal glands. The superolateral portion of the right kidney is adjacent to the liver, and the inferior portion is adjacent to the hepatic flexure of the colon. The superolateral anterior border of the left kidney is near the spleen, with its medial aspect adjacent to the stomach and the inferior portion adjacent to the colon. Posteriorly, the kidneys are close to the inferior portions of the diaphragm and lie adjacent to the psoas muscles. The inferior vena cava lies near the right

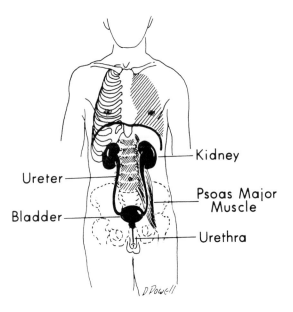

Fig. 9-1.
  Anatomical relationships of the kidneys to other structures.

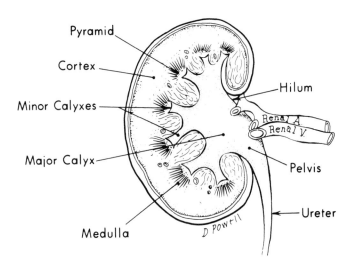

Fig. 9-2.
  Gross renal anatomy (coronal view).

kidney, being interposed between the aorta and the kidney. The kidneys are generally not fixed to the abdominal wall and are noted to move with respiratory effort.

The ureters are tubular structures which move the urine from the kidneys to the urinary bladder. The area where the renal pelvis joins the ureter is called the *ureteropelvic junction.* The ureter courses down over the psoas muscles and enters the pelvis just lateral to the sacroiliac joint and then courses posteriorly before entering the inferior aspect of the urinary bladder. In its upper portion, the duodenal loop is in proximity to the right ureter; and as the ureter courses inferiorly it crosses the hypogastric or external iliac vessel. The left ureter is also in proximity to the spermatic artery.

The urinary bladder is located in the pelvis, posterior to the symphysis pubis and anterior to the rectosigmoid colon, with the female uterus separating the bladder from the colon. The size and shape of the bladder vary in proportion to the amount of urine present. Care should be taken in interpreting pressure defects in or on an undistended bladder.

Indications for doing an intravenous urogram are many but can be classified into the following: (1) obstruction, (2) abnormal urinary sediment, (3) arterial hypertension, and (4) localization of abdominal masses.

CLINICAL RELATIONSHIPS

Symptoms referable to the urinary tract are generally not noted on the routine physical examination but are usually suspected on the basis of examination of urine or blood specimens. The indications for routine examination of blood or urine specimens or both are therefore obvious. There may be some clinical indications, however, of urinary tract abnormalities. Pain occurring along the course of the ureter may be referred to the groins. Typical renal pain in the costovertebral region is usually dull and aching and occurs generally in severe kidney infection, hydronephrosis, and in large kidney tumors or infarcts. Renal colic is severe renal pain which is sharp and agonizing and refers along the course of the ureter toward the genital and loin region. It is highlighted by paroxysmal attacks between which a constant low-grade pain may be felt in the groin area. Occasionally there may be tenderness in the costovertebral area which may be elicited by palpation with the blunt portion of the fist, and on occasion there is fullness in the costovertebral region secondary to a perinephric abscess or renal mass. An important differential sign in separating renal from biliary colic is that renal colic rarely ever refers pain to the subscapular area as contrasted to biliary colic.

The discovery of abnormal urine by the patient because of its odor, volume, color, or pain on micturition is one of the more common signs relating to the genitourinary tract. Gross or microscopical hematuria generally indicates the presence of urinary calculus, tumor, or, occasionally, tuberculosis or pyelone-phritis. The importance of obtaining an adequate clean urine specimen cannot be overemphasized.

Change in renal function as reflected clinically varies with the degree to which the kidneys may react to compensate for decreased function in one or both kid-neys. As renal reserve decreases, the patient may exhibit fatigue, headache, anorexia, mild changes in blood pressure, and anemia. Edema may be present in later stages. With an acute decrease in renal function, the urine output is usually diminished to a mild degree and then may increase to polyuria as the patient's disease becomes chronic. As renal function further decreases, uremia may develop which is generally the intensification of the symptoms of decreased renal function. During this time the patient may become restless and have mental changes. The skin may become dry and turgid, with sensory changes, hypertension, and generalized edema present. Terminally, the patient may pro-ceed to convulsions. Typical edematous changes may occur in the colon, small bowel, pericardium, and lung fields, as shown roentgenographically.

Previous mention was made of the anatomical relationships of the kidneys and surrounding structures. Knowledge of this anatomy may be utilized in locating probable abdominal masses not related to the genitourinary tract. For example, the presence of a nonrenal mass displacing the right kidney laterally and inferiorly would be suspected of being duodenal, biliary, adrenal, or hepatic in origin. Displacement of the ureter or bladder may be indicative of tumors originating from pelvic organs. Anterior or lateral or anterior and lateral dis-placement of the ureters may be seen in lymph node enlargement from lymphoma.

One of the newer uses of urograms in patient evaluation is for the study of surgically correctable renal vascular hypertension. The minute-sequence urogram performed by rapid injection of contrast material and rapid-filming sequences demonstrating the nephrogram and excretory functions of the kidney as related to its size is an accurate indication of abnormal renal blood flow. Renal size 2 cm less than the opposite kidney, asymmetric appearance of a nephrogram, or excretory phase differential between the kidneys are the more reliable indi-cations of decreased renal blood flow. Renovascular hypertension rarely occurs in the adult Negro male, and this should be considered when requesting such an examination. The finding of an abnormal minute-sequence phenomenon may lead one to request renal arteriograms or a renogram to better visualize the renal artery and renal arterial flow.

ROENTGENOGRAPHIC CONSIDERATIONS

Examination of the urinary tract should be preceded by a plain film of the abdomen to demonstrate the renal shadows and pelvis adequately (Fig. 9-3). With modern technique using high-volume contrast material, it is no longer

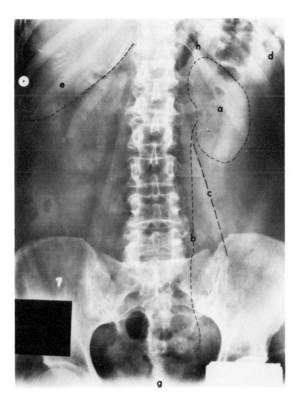

Fig. 9-3.

    Plain roentgenogram taken prior to an intravenous urogram. Notice the renal shadows adjacent to the psoas stripes. a, renal outline; b, ureter; c, psoas stripe; d, location of spleen; e, location of liver and gallbladder; f, properitoneal fat stripe; g, region of bladder; h, region of stomach.

mandatory that the patient be dehydrated, although the bowel should be adequately cleansed of feces and gas so that the renal shadows can be visualized. Normally the kidney shadows are fairly well demonstrated by the presence of the perinephric fat if they lie in their normal location adjacent to the L-2 or L-1 vertebral bodies. The inferior poles are slightly deviated laterally. The psoas shadows should be sharp, although if previous infection has been present, some obliteration of the psoas shadows may be noted which may not be indicative of active disease. There should be no obvious calcific densities overlying the renal shadows or course of the ureters. If such densities are present, proper oblique films should be obtained before the injection of contrast material for comparative studies with subsequent films.

    Filming sequence of urograms varies from hospital to hospital, but generally there is a film taken shortly after the injection of the contrast material, one film some 10 minutes later, and one taken 15 to 20 minutes after injection of the contrast material. On the initial film there is usually a good nephrogram effect demonstrating the renal outline (Fig. 9-4). The calyceal system usually presents as buttercup-shaped projections surrounding the renal papillae. The cupping of the calyx should be sharp, and there should be good filling of the calyxes. The renal pelvis is generally well demarcated; and if an adequate amount of contrast is used, there is also fairly good demonstration of the ureters all the way to the bladder. Delayed films usually show normal bladder distention, outlining a

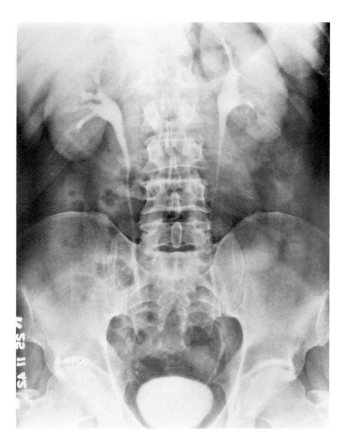

Fig. 9-4.

Normal intravenous urogram. Notice the symmetry of the renal shadows and delicacy of the calyxes. Occasionally a bump may be seen in the renal outline due to fetal lobulation, which is a normal variant. The ureters course medially over the psoas muscles before crossing the sacrum and entering the pelvis. The bladder is well filled with contrast media. Compare to Figures 9-1 and 9-2.

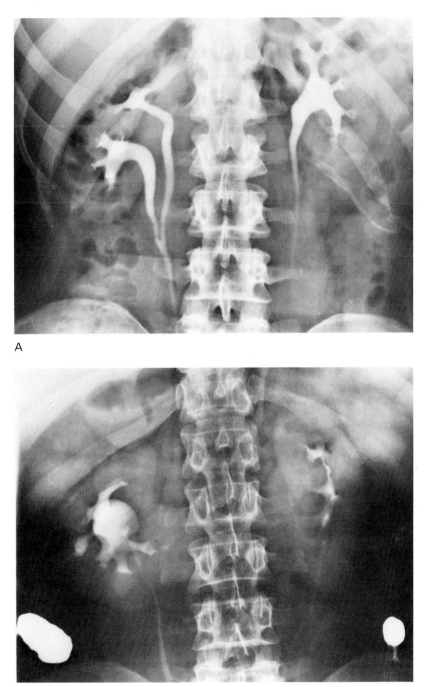

A

B

Figure 9-5.
(Legend on page 193.)

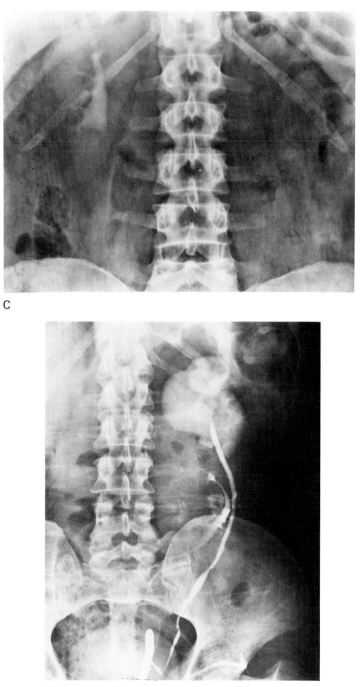

C

D

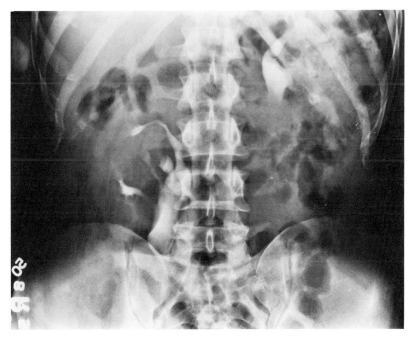

E

Fig. 9-5.

Some common anomalies seen on urograms. (A) Double right renal pelvis. (B) Horseshoe kidney variant. Notice how the inferior poles of the kidneys are rotated inward and the malposition of the renal pelves with partial ureteropelvic obstruction on the right. Any number of variations of the amount of tissue connecting the lower poles may be seen.

(C) Congenital absence of the left kidney. An amputated lower rib may be seen in patients following nephrectomy. (D) Fused, crossed ectopia with ureteropelvic obstruction of the upper kidney. (E) Ectopic right kidney (pelvic kidney). Three aberrant vessels were found supplying this kidney.

smooth bladder wall with no evidence of displacement. The film taken after voiding is valuable in the male for estimating residual urine.

Congenital Variations in the Kidney. Some of the more common congenital findings (Fig. 9-5) include double collecting systems, renal ectopia, nephroptosis (floating kidney), and occasionally horseshoe kidney variations. The duplicated collecting system presents as a double renal pelvis and ureter leading from a fused single kidney, although on occasion a completely duplicated kidney may be present. In renal ectopia, the kidney shadow is not in its normal location and may, for example, be located in the pelvis rather than in its normal position. Particularly in some lean and athletic persons, the kidney may be extremely mobile according to the position of the patient and will fall toward the pelvis when the patient is in the upright position.

Kidney Obstruction. The obstructive pattern is demonstrated by a delayed function of the affected kidney or kidneys and is seen roentgenographically by delayed function and an increased nephrogram phase as compared to the opposite kidney (Fig. 9-6) and later by dilatation of the calyxes (calicectasis) or renal pelvis (pyelectasis), with the dilatation of the combined ureter, pelvis, and calyxes termed *hydronephrosis.*

The obstructive pattern (Fig. 9-7) also is caused by such conditions as an aberrant vessel crossing the ureteropelvic junction and producing obstruction of the pelvis, with subsequent dilatation of the pelvis and related calicectasis. It should be pointed out that there may be marked pyelectasis, particularly with associated extrarenal pelves, with very little calicectasis. In addition, calculi and renal

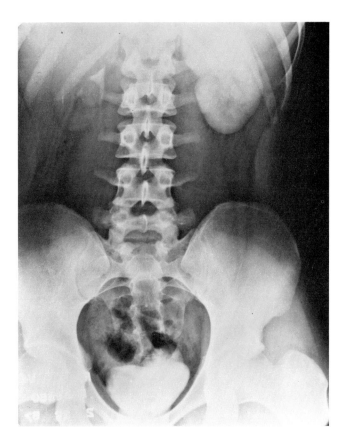

Fig. 9-6.
  Delayed and prominent nephrogram of left kidney due to obstruction of the distal ureter by a calculus.

tumors may obstruct the outflow tract from the renal pelvis, producing the same effect. Obstructions in the ureter occurring anywhere along its course are most commonly caused by calculi. There is associated dilatation of the ureter down to the point of obstruction. Occasionally ureteral tumors may produce the same effect. The presence of diverticula, particularly at the ureterovesical junction, may also produce obstruction. In patients with previous inflammatory disease in the retroperitoneal fascial plane, subsequent fibrosis of the tissue surrounding the ureter may produce obstruction, generally at the level of the false pelvic inlet. Stricture of the ureter secondary to inflammatory disease or operative manipulation may produce localized obstruction. Congenital causes such as the lack of ganglionic cells in the ureter may lead to such conditions as megaureter and abnormal location of the ureter, such as behind the vena cava, which may also produce obstruction.

In some patients, incompetence of the ureteral valve as it enters the vesicular musculature may allow reflux of the urine back up into the ureter, with resultant dilatation of either one or both ureters (Fig. 9-8A). The presence of a pelvic mass may produce extrinsic pressure upon either or both ureters, causing the same effect. One of the more common pelvic masses is an enlarging uterus due to fibroids or pregnancy, with subsequent pressure on the ureter and partial or sometimes complete obstruction. In the older male, one of the most common causes of obstruction of the bladder neck outlet is enlargement of the prostate gland (Fig. 9-8B). In some patients, the presence of valves within the bladder neck or fibrous bands or bars within the urethra may cause outlet obstruction.

Changes in the buttercup appearance of the calyxes may indicate a disease process within the renal substance (Fig. 9-9). Blunted calyxes are usually typical of pyelonephritis; and distortion or displacement of the calyxes may be seen in renal tumors, infection, cysts, trauma, and other modalities. Renal cysts (Fig. 9-10) and tumors (Fig. 9-11) may enlarge sufficiently to distort the outline of the kidney. It should be noted that the urogram taken only in the AP or PA plane may not demonstrate distortion or displacement of posterior calyxes which could possibly be demonstrated better on oblique films or with nephrotomography. In differentiating renal cysts from renal mass lesions, a nephrotomogram may show a well-demarcated lesion with no nephrogram phase in cysts which may be a differential point in excluding renal cysts from renal tumors.

The presence of calcification within renal masses is also a differential point. Hypernephromas generally do not calcify unless they are large and necrotic and are usually seen in older patients. Children having Wilms' tumor reveal a renal mass without appreciable calcification. The same type of lesion may be seen in a neuroblastoma; but in this case, there is rather marked calcification.

To summarize, distortion of the collecting system anatomy may lead one to suspect the presence of a pathological condition. Obviously, some disease

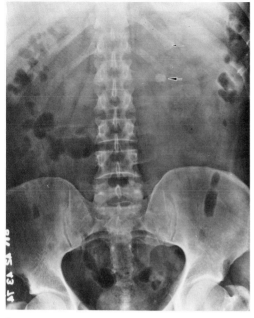

A

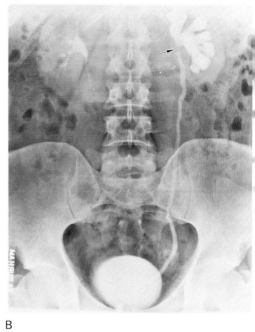

B

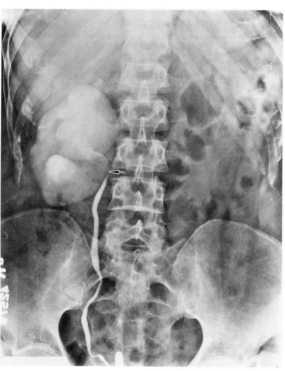

C

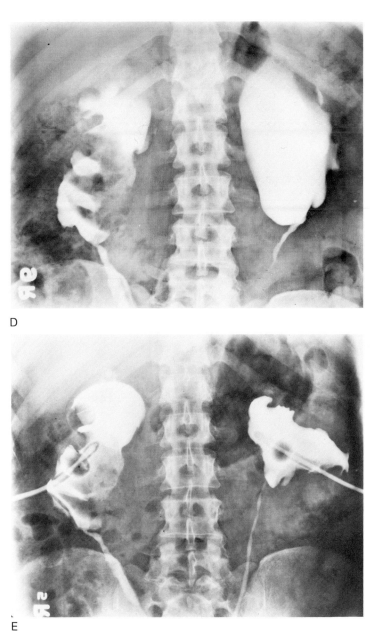

D

E

Fig. 9-7.

The *obstructive pattern* implies some degree of resistance to the outflow of urine.

(A, B) Laminated stone in the region of the left kidney seen on the plain film. (Notice also the amputated ribs from previous surgery.) The urogram (B) demonstrates dilatation of the calyxes proximal to the stone in addition to partial obstruction of the left ureter at the ureterovesical junction.

(C) Retrograde urogram demonstrating marked ureteropelvic obstruction (arrow) secondary to an aberrant vessel.

(D, E) Bilateral ureteropelvic obstruction in a horseshoe kidney variant. Notice how the ureters exit inferiorly, typical of horseshoe kidneys. This patient was treated by inserting drains into the kidneys (nephrostomies).

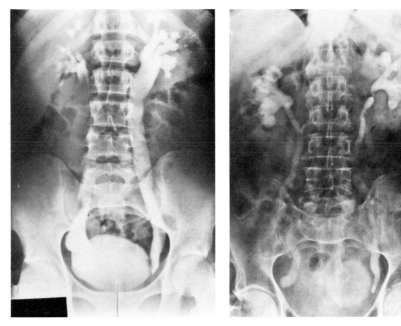

A   B

Fig. 9-8.

(A) Bilateral hydronephrosis secondary to ureteral reflux and pyelonephritis. (B) Bilateral hydronephrosis secondary to bladder neck obstruction. Notice the large bladder diverticulum presenting as an ovoid density overlying the left side of the bladder.

processes produce such subtle changes that follow-up examinations for comparison must be obtained. This is particularly true in patients with occult microscopical hematuria which may be coming from a small hypernephroma not visualized either by renal scan, nephrotomograms, or renal arteriography. In addition, when requesting the urogram one must also inform the radiologist of a suspected abdominal mass lesion so that appropriate across-table films may be obtained to demonstrate any significant anterior deviation of the ureters.

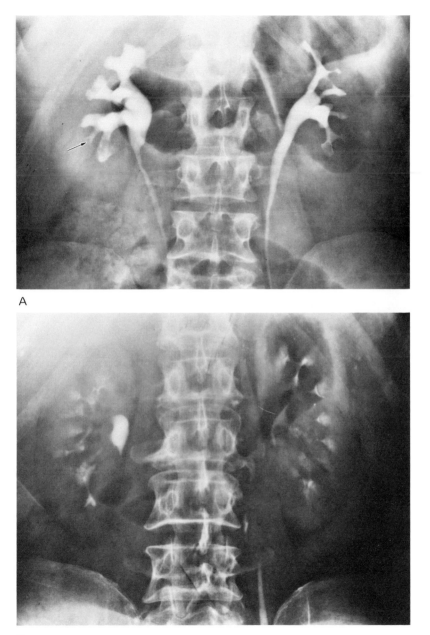

A

B

Figure 9-9.
(Legend on page 201.)

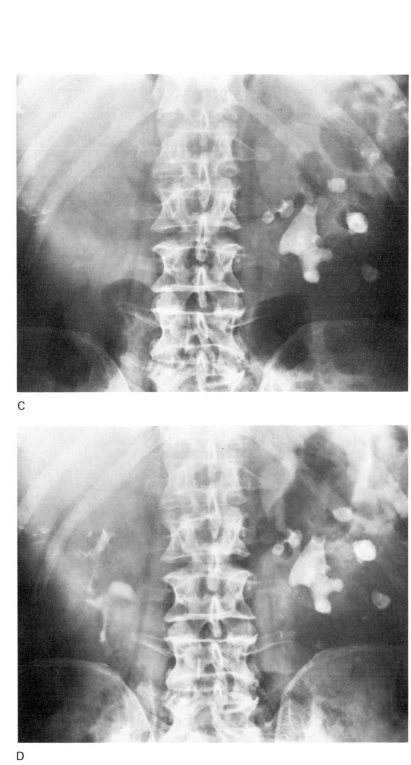

C

D

200

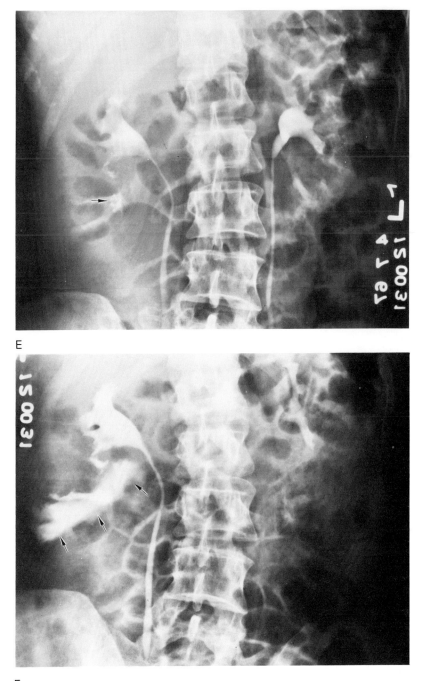

E

F

Fig. 9-9.

(A) Blunted calyxes secondary to chronic pyelonephritis. On the right a single normal calyx (arrow) is present. (B) Medullary sponge kidney demonstrating dilated distal tubules. The dilated tubules appear as rays emanating from the calyx.

(C, D) Staghorn calculus, plain film (C) and urogram (D). There is very poor renal function on the left.

(E, F) Traumatic rupture, right kidney. The urogram (E) demonstrates a peculiar collection of contrast media in the lower pole. The retrograde study (F) creates a higher than physiological pressure in the renal collecting system, forcing the contrast media out of its normal channels.

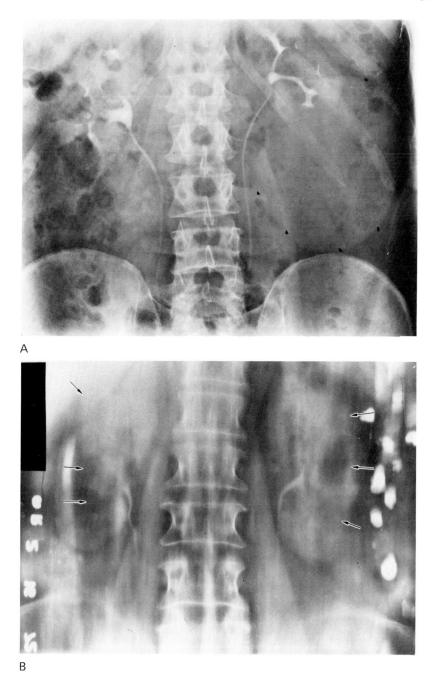

A

B

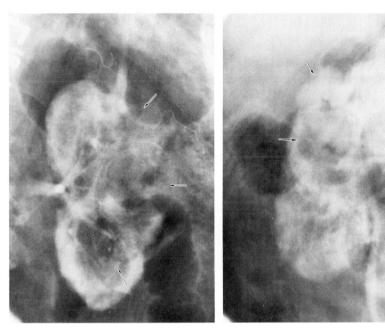

C   D

Fig. 9-10.

(A) Large renal cyst projecting from the lower pole of the left kidney.

(B, C, D) Multiple small cysts suspected on the urogram (not shown) with multiple defects shown on the tomogram (B) and demonstrated conclusively on the angiogram (D).

Cystograms. On most occasions the urinary bladder is adequately visualized during the process of performing an intravenous urogram. At times the bladder is evaluated directly by means of a cystogram. The cystogram is performed by insertion of a catheter through the urethra and filling the bladder with contrast material. The bladder must be filled slowly or bladder spasm will occur and prevent adequate distention.

Infections involving the upper urinary tract also involve the bladder. Considering that vesicular papillomas found in the bladder are premalignant tumors, the bladder is one of the most common places for urinary tract tumors. Such things as bladder calculi, diverticuli, bladder neck obstruction, congenital anomalies, trauma, and infection may be evaluated by means of a cystogram (Fig. 9-12).

One of the more frequent reasons for obtaining a cystogram is to identify vesicoureteral reflux. As the ureters insert through the bladder wall, they diagonally transverse the muscle layers of the wall; and as the bladder distends,

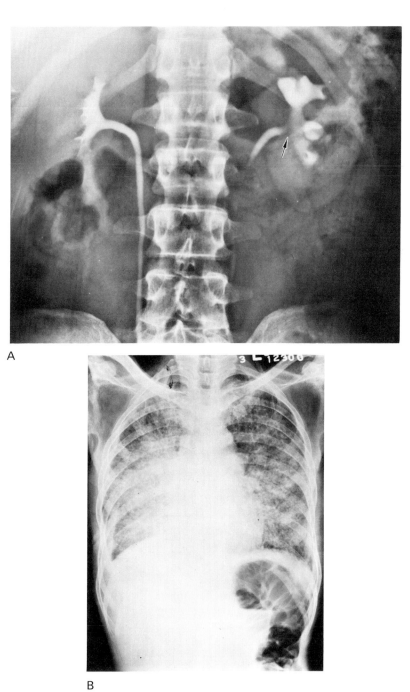

A

B

Figure 9-11.
(Legend on page 206.)

204

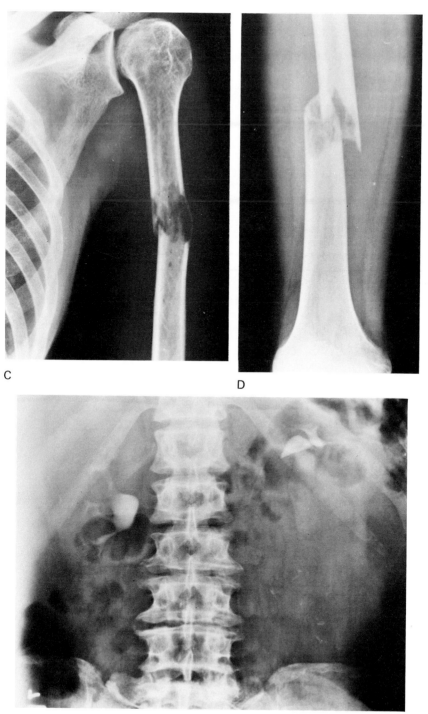

C

D

E

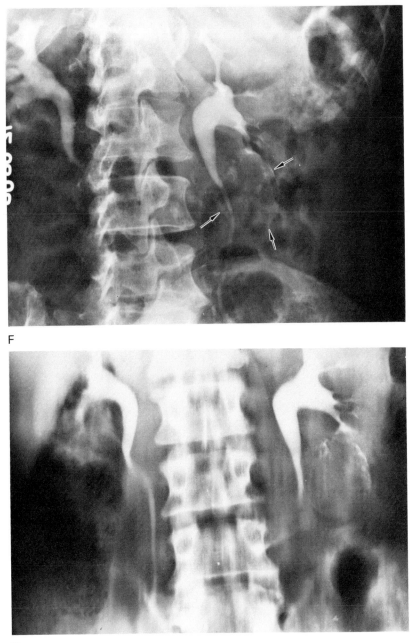

F

G

Fig. 9-11.

(A–D) Hypernephroma with minor changes, left calyxes (A), but with widespread metastases. The urogram (A) was performed almost one year after the other films were taken. The fractures (C, D) are pathological.

(E) Large hypernephroma, left kidney, displacing kidney upward and extending almost to the pelvic brim.

(F, G) Hypernephroma extending from the lower pole of the left kidney; seen better on the tomogram (G).

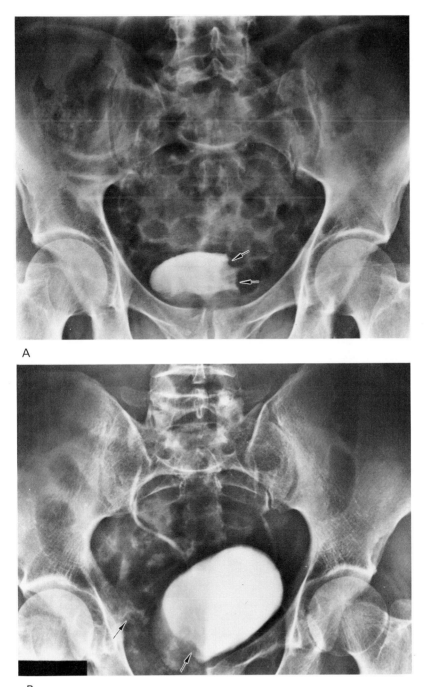

A

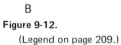

B

Figure 9-12.
(Legend on page 209.)

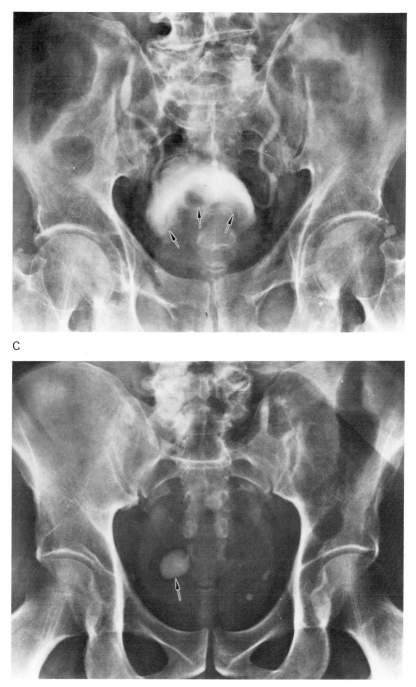

C

D

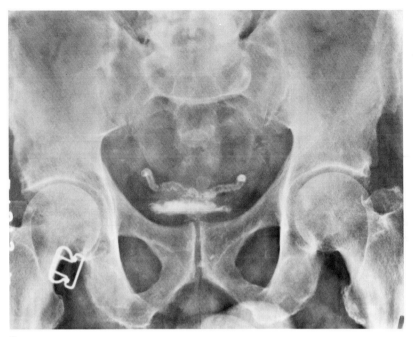

E

Fig. 9-12.
Various bladder conditions. (A) Transitional cell carcinoma of the bladder. Patient was asymptomatic five weeks prior to admission. He exhibited sudden onset of painless, total hematuria. (B) Chondrosarcoma of right pubic ramus displacing bladder. The entire pubic ramus has been destroyed by the tumor. (C) Carcinoma of prostate gland invading base of bladder. (D) Bladder stone removed at cystoscopy. The other densities are phleboliths. (E) Calcification of vas deferens and seminal vesicles in a diabetic patient.

pressure on the muscle layers of the bladder wall produce an effective valving effect to prevent urine from refluxing from the bladder into the ureter. If bladder infection occurs and the ureteral "valve" is incompetent, infected urine may reflux into the ureter and kidney, producing inflammation in those areas. In order to demonstrate reflux, the cystogram must be performed prior to an intravenous study. As one would imagine, if an intravenous study were performed first, one could not determine if contrast media noted in the ureter(s) had refluxed from below or had been excreted normally from above.

Urethrograms. Examination of the urethra (Fig. 9-13) is accomplished by a voiding cystourethrogram; following a cystogram, an x-ray exposure is made while the patient is urinating. This view effectively demonstrates the bladder neck and urethra under physiological pressures. On occasion, retrograde

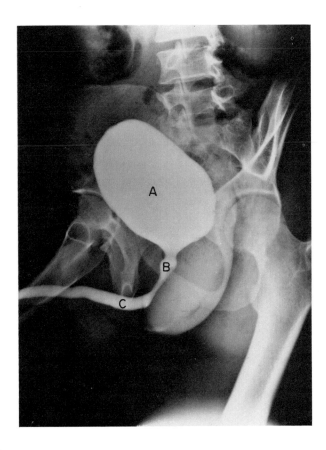

Fig. 9-13.
Normal male voiding cystourethrogram. A, bladder; B, prostatic urethra; C, urethra.

urethrograms are performed when a cystogram is not necessary. This study is done by simply injecting contrast media from a syringe through the urethra into the bladder. Retrograde urethrograms are generally used to follow the course of urethral strictures.

Other Examinations. The preceding paragraphs emphasize the urogram as the main examination for study of the kidneys, ureters, and bladder. Other procedures are also important in radiology and urology and often contribute clinical information when a urogram is not possible. The antegrade urogram is obtained by directly instilling contrast material through a draining catheter. This examination is useful for evaluation of renal emptying following nephrostomy, ileal conduits, and so on. Retrograde pyelography is not as commonly used today as it was prior to the introduction of drip infusion pyelography. Such studies may be indicated, however, to evaluate a suspicious lesion noted on the urogram or, if a patient is in renal failure, to demonstrate patency of at least one ureter.

READING LIST

Emmett, J. *Clinical Urography.* Philadelphia: Saunders, 1964.
Meschan, I. (Ed.). The Urinary Tract. *Radiol. Clin. North Am.* vol. 3, no. 1, 1965.
Ney, C., and Friedenburg, R. M. *Radiographic Atlas of the Genitourinary System.* Philadelphia: Lippincott, 1966.
Thornbury, J. R., and Culp, D. A. *The Urinary Tract.* Chicago: Year Book, 1967.

The Lungs and Mediastinum   **10**

IN THE EARLY HOURS of the morning some years ago a sleepy radiology resident was discussing with a medical resident the urgent need for a routine chest x-ray. After much hassle, the medical resident blurted, "We don't examine the chest anymore; we take a chest film to see if anything is wrong!" Although there is some serious doubt as to the entire validity of that statement, our clinical colleagues have come to rely heavily upon the chest roentgenogram as a screening device for anatomical variations of the thorax and for subtle pathological changes.

The chest roentgenogram probably contains more bits of information than films of any other region of the body. Indeed, the chest is perhaps the most complex portion of the body examined roentgenographically. In order to appreciate the complexity of a chest roentgenogram, the student should have at least a good, sound working knowledge of the anatomical relationships of the different organs located within the thorax. Only by understanding these relationships in conjunction with clinical information does a chest roentgenogram prove useful.

ANATOMY OF THE CHEST FILM

The chest film contains information referable to the thorax and as such demonstrates the soft tissues of the thoracic wall, the bony structures, upper portion of the abdomen, the diaphragm, lower portions of the neck, the mediastinum (including the heart), and the lungs. The cardiac silhouette and great vessels which are contained within the mediastinum are discussed in Chapter 11, The Heart and Great Vessels. The significant areas of interest are noted in Figure 10-1.

213

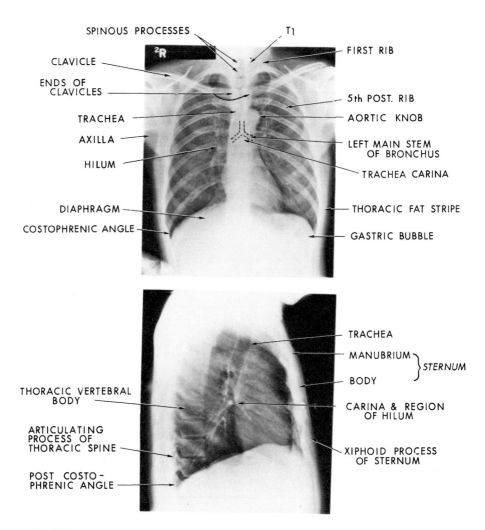

Fig. 10-1.
   Labeled posteroanterior and lateral chest films.

Soft Tissues

The excess or diminution of thoracic soft tissues indicates a pathological process, either past or present. Normally one may see the lateral thoracic fat stripe as a thin, radiolucent line along the side of the chest, extending from the axilla down to the level of the pelvic brim. Fat deposition in the supraclavicular areas may also be seen. Excessive cutaneous fluid such as from edema secondary to heart failure may obliterate the stripes. Infiltration or change in the fatty tissue by collagen diseases may make the fat deposition roentgenographically imperceptible. Enlargement of lymph nodes in the axilla or supraclavicular areas may force expansion of the fatty tissue into a mass effect. An obese person may have obvious enlargement of soft tissue as seen lateral to the bony thorax.

On most chest films, the pectoral muscle groups appear as veils extending over a moderate portion of the upper lateral thorax. Enlargement of the pectoral muscle as, for example, by persons doing hard physical labor such as lifting will accentuate this appearance and should be recognized as a normal variant rather than a pathological process. If a person does mostly right-arm or hand labor, there may be a unilateral enlargement of that muscle group. Differentiation from a chest mass usually poses no problem, since the edge of the muscle group can generally be noted extending out of the lung shadow.

Breasts, both in the male and the female, cast homogeneous shadows over the midchest and are prominent in some persons and inconspicuous in others. The absence of a breast shadow in the female must be noted, since the primary assumption is that the breast was surgically removed because of carcinoma. Concomitant absence of axillary soft tissues usually indicates a radical mastectomy for carcinoma of the breast. Nipples are more prominent in some persons than others and often create the appearance of a lung nodule. The bilateral symmetrical location of nipples is normally at the level of the fourth or fifth anterior rib space and is useful in differentiating nipple shadows from other possible chest lesions. Generally if one nipple is noticeable, the other is also seen. On occasion the nipples must be marked with a piece of lead or other metallic material and roentgenograms obtained to differentiate between nipple shadows and possible lung lesions. One should not fall into the trap of obtaining only PA films, since on occasion a pulmonary nodule may be hidden in a nipple shadow. Stereoscopic chest films are usually better for this type of examination.

When requesting a chest film, the examiner should note the presence of soft tissue densities located on the chest wall. Enlarged moles, warts, fibrolipomas, and other such surface lesions may present as a pulmonary density and lead to a confusing diagnosis.

At least a portion of the upper abdomen should be included on all chest films. Note should be made as to the location of the gastric air bubble in relation to the left hemidiaphragm, the presence of calcific densities in the region of the gallbladder or kidney, and any possible enlargement of the spleen or liver. On occasion a mass within the gastric air bubble may lead to a diagnosis of carcinoma of the stomach, made from a routine chest film.

Bony Thorax

The reader is referred to the Appendix to refresh his memory concerning the bony structures of the chest. To reiterate, the chest film demonstrates the ribs, thoracic and lower cervical spines, and the sternum. One should be aware of the technique used in obtaining the films, since high-kilovoltage film technique does not adequately demonstrate bony trabecular pattern; and if a bony abnormality is suspected, properly exposed films using bone technique should be obtained. On most properly exposed films, however, sufficient bone detail is present to allow one to recognize bony abnormalities (Fig. 10-2).

One should develop the habit of locating lesions according to rib level, designating whether the rib is posterior or anterior. Generally it is better to count from the first rib downward, rather than from the twelfth rib upward, since all too often one cannot detect the lower ribs through the abdominal soft tissue densities. Proper film exposure should dictate that the examiner be able to view the lower thoracic spine through the heart shadow, and some observers believe that the film should be dark enough that one can see the disk space.

Lungs

There is one lung in each hemithorax, with the two lungs being separated by the contents of the mediastinum. On the right the lung is subdivided into three lobes; namely, the upper, middle, and lower; on the left only two lobes are present, the upper and the lower.

Separating lobes one from another are interleaved portions of visceral pleura called *fissures*. The right major fissure separates the upper and middle lobes from the lower lobe. The left major fissure separates the upper lobe from the lower lobe. Separating the right upper and middle lobes is the minor fissure, composed again of visceral pleura. Anatomically, a minor fissure is not seen on the left except in a small percentage of cases in which a fissure does exist between the upper lobe and lingula. Accessory fissures such as the azygos fissure in the right upper lobe and the inferior accessory fissure separating the medial basal segment of the right lower lobe from the remainder of the right lower lobe may also be noted.

The major fissures are not seen on the PA film, since the thickness of the pleura is insufficient to absorb enough radiation to allow a shadow to be cast on the x-ray film. On the lateral film, the major fissure can usually be seen separating the different lobes. This fissure appears as a long, oblique, thin line beginning at the level of T-4 or T-5 and coursing anteriorly to intersect the anterior chest at the inferior cardiopulmonary region. However, the minor

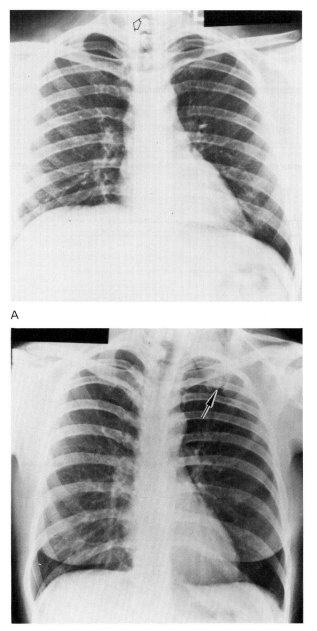

Fig. 10-2.

Normal chest films, with the exception of: (A) metastatic sarcoma to the right lower cervical spine; (B) Sprengel's deformity of the left scapula with omovertebral joint.

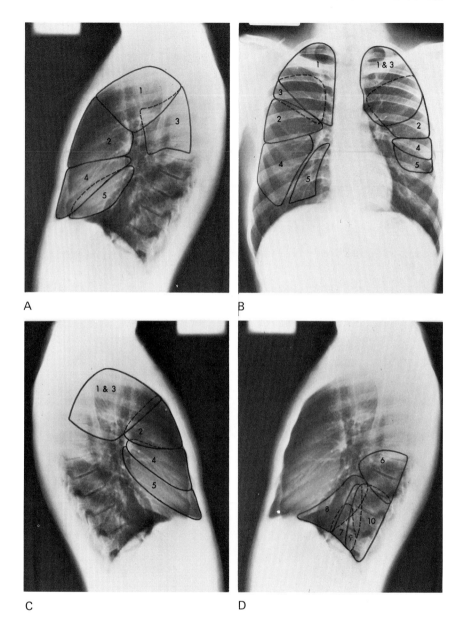

A

B

C

D

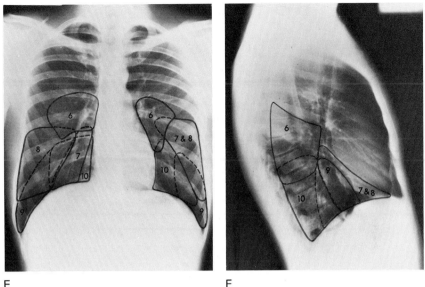

E   F

Fig. 10-3.

Approximate location of the bronchopulmonary segments.

R U L
{
1. Apical
2. Anterior
3. Posterior

R M L
{
4. Lateral
5. Medial

R L L
{
6. Superior
7. Medial basal
8. Anterior basal
9. Lateral basal
10. Posterior basal

L U L
{
1 & 3. Apical posterior
2. Anterior
4. Superior lingula
5. Inferior lingula

L L L
{
6. Superior
7 & 8. Anteromedial basal
9. Lateral basal
10. Posterior basal

RUL = right upper lobe; RML = right middle lobe; RLL = right lower lobe; LUL = left upper lobe; LLL = left lower lobe.

fissure separating the middle from the upper lobe on the right can generally be seen on both the PA and the lateral films. On the PA film it is in the midportion of the chest, extending laterally from the hilar region. On the lateral film it appears as a white line beginning at the midportion of the major fissure and coursing anteriorly to the chest wall. If a fissure does occur between the lingula and upper lobe of the left lung, it is in the same position as the minor fissure on the opposite side.

Bronchopulmonary Segments. Each lobe of the lung is subdivided into broncho-pulmonary segments (Fig. 10-3). On the right, the upper lobe is subdivided into three pulmonary segments, namely the apical, anterior, and posterior. The middle lobe is subdivided into lateral and medial segments, and the lower lobe is divided into superior, medial basal, anterior basal, lateral basal, and posterior basal segments.

On the left, the upper lobe demonstrates fused apical and posterior segments and is termed the *apical posterior segment,* with an anterior segment similar to that on the right. The inferior part of the upper lobe is called the *lingula* and is subdivided into superior and inferior portions. The lower lobe has only four segments, with the anterior and medial segments fused into the anteromedial basal segments; and there are also the superior, lateral basal, and posterior basal segments.

In viewing the chest roentgenogram, one must visualize the pulmonary segments in three dimensions or one will have difficulty in placing the exact location of pathological processes. Both the PA and lateral films must be utilized to recognize the location of each segment. Even though Figure 10-3 demonstrates the approximate location of the bronchopulmonary segments, a narrative has always been useful to the inexperienced individual.

The apical segment lies in the uppermost portion of the lung and is generally superior and medial to the second anterior rib, extending from the upper lateral thoracic wall to the mediastinum; on the lateral film it overlies the axilla. The posterior segment of the upper lobe involves the lateral chest wall and tapers toward the mediastinum and on the lateral film is noted to be posterior, overlying the spine. This is contrasted to the anterior segment of the upper lobe, which on the lateral film is anterior and superior to the heart and minor fissure and on the anterior film shows more encroachment upon the mediastinum.

The lateral segment of the middle lobe, as the name implies, is noted to be lateral on the anterior chest and involves the thoracic wall but spares the mediastinum and costophrenic angle. On the lateral film, this segment occupies the region where the major and minor fissures bisect. The medial portion of the middle lobe is anterior and obliterates the mediastinum and adjacent heart border and overlies the anterior heart on the lateral film.

The superior segment of the lower lobe is located in the same general area as the anterior segment on the PA film but encroaches more upon the mediastinum. It generally is at the level of the hilum; and on the lateral film it is noted to be posterior, just beneath the uppermost margin of the major fissure. The medial basal and posterior basal segments overlap each other on the PA film, but on the lateral film the posterior segment overlies the spine and the medial basal segment overlies the paracardiac area just behind the cardiac silhouette. The anterior basal segment is located slightly lateral to the cardiac silhouette on the PA film and on the lateral film overlies the cardiac silhouette. The anterior basal segment does not occupy the costophrenic angle. The lateral basal segment, as the name implies, involves the costophrenic angle and on the lateral film obscures the region of the medial basal segment.

The left lung demonstrates essentially the same segmental distribution except that the apical and posterior segments of the left upper lobe are fused and present as one segment. There is no middle lobe on the left, but a corresponding area termed the *lingula* is present. Instead of being divided into medial and lateral segments, the lingula is divided into superior and inferior segments. The segments of the left lower lobe are essentially the same as those of the right lower lobe, with the exception that the anterior and medial basal segments are fused.

Trachea and Bronchi. Distributing air to the pulmonary segments are bronchi named for the pulmonary segments which they serve (Fig. 10-4). The main air channel is the trachea, which begins at the level of the epiglottis in the midline. In children there is a tendency for the trachea to buckle as the patient moves his head, but in the adult this is generally a fixed structure and does not move appreciably with movement of the head. At the level of T-5 the trachea divides into right and left bronchi, with the acute angle at the bifurcation termed the *carina.* The left main-stem bronchus divides into the upper and lower lobe bronchi. Immediately after the takeoff of the upper lobe bronchus on the left there is a division into smaller-ordered bronchi going to the lingula. In the right lung immediately after the bifurcation there is a major division given off to the upper lobe. From the takeoff of the right upper lobe to the further subdivision of bronchi is termed the *bronchus intermedius.* Coming off posteriorly from the bronchus intermedius is the bronchus to the superior segment of the lower lobe. At about the same level, the bronchus to the middle lobe is given off.

One of the major difficulties in determining abnormalities of the trachea and major bronchi is the occlusion or absence of one bronchus. For example, a small tumor may occlude one bronchus, and at bronchography or tomography this occluded bronchus may be overlooked. One should develop the habit of positively identifying each bronchus.

Pulmonary Blood Supply. The lungs are supplied by two different sets of blood vessels, the pulmonary and the bronchial arteries. The pulmonary artery transports venous blood from the right ventricle and distributes it to the right and left pulmonary arteries (Fig. 10-5A). The right pulmonary artery courses behind the ascending aorta and superior vena cava and in front of the right bronchus. It gives off two major branches, one to the lower lobe and one to the upper and middle lobes. The left main-stem pulmonary artery courses in front of the descending aorta and the left main-stem bronchus. It gives off two branches, one to the upper lobe and one to the lower lobe. Generally one branch supplies one segment, although small branches from adjacent arteries may supply small areas of adjacent segments.

Coursing in the same interstitium as the pulmonary arteries are the pulmonary veins, which transport oxygenated blood to the left atrium and on the chest film occupy positions slightly inferior to the pulmonary arteries (see Fig. 10-5B).

The second primary blood supply to the lung is that of the bronchial arteries, which supply nutrients for cellular metabolism. Generally there is one bronchial

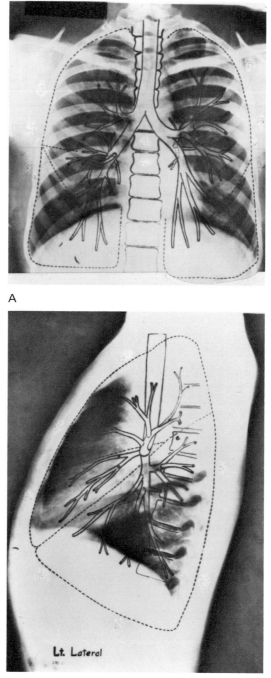

A

B

Lt. Lateral

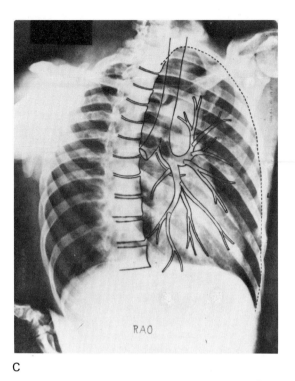

C

Fig. 10-4.
    Approximate location of the trachea and major bronchi in relation to the lung fields:
(A) posteroanterior; (B) left lateral; (C) right anterior oblique.

artery on the right with two on the left, all arising from the anterior portion
of the thoracic aorta or, occasionally, singularly from the upper intercostal
arteries.

Hilum. The confluence of the major bronchi and vessels at the root of the lung
is called the *hilum.* Roentgenographically, the hilum is composed primarily of
vascular shadows (see Fig. 10-5). On the PA film the left hilum is slightly higher
than the right, but occasionally both hila are at the same level. A rule of thumb
is that the right hilum should never be higher than the left, and a pathological
process is suspected when it is. On the lateral chest film there is general superimposition of the hila, with the left hilum slightly more posterior than the right.
The lymph nodes draining the lungs are in these areas, and the radiologist must
take care lest subtle enlargement of a lymph node merging with vascular
shadows be overlooked.

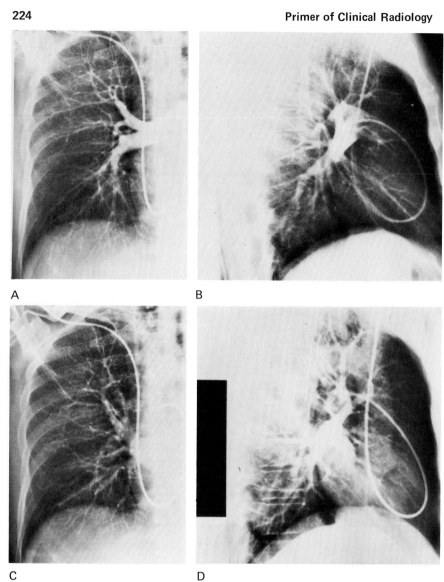

Fig. 10-5.

Normal pulmonary angiogram demonstrating (A) pulmonary artery, (B) lateral pulmonary artery, (C) pulmonary vein, (D) lateral pulmonary vein. Notice that the arteries are located superiorly to the veins.

Diaphragm

The diaphragm is a peculiar musculofibrous septum separating the thoracic from the abdominal cavity. In the normal person the right hemidiaphragm is 1 to 2 cm higher than the left. There is about a 3 cm average movement between full inspiration and forced expiration. The height of the diaphragm constantly varies with the degree of inspiration or expiration and also according to the volume of the abdominal organs. With the patient recumbent, abdominal pressure raises the level of the diaphragm and obscures the lower lung fields.

It is common to see elevation of the left hemidiaphragm due to gaseous distention of the stomach or splenic flexure of the colon (Fig. 10-6). One or both segments of the diaphragm may be elevated due to phrenic nerve paresis. Loss of lung volume, scoliosis, obesity, and rotation are other factors affecting diaphragmatic height.

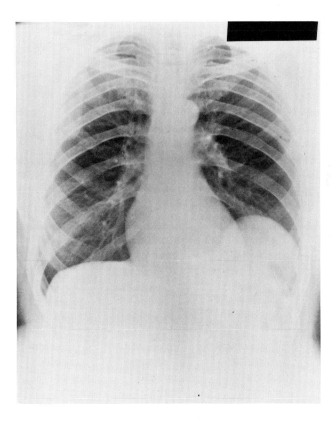

Fig. 10-6.
Physiological elevation of the left hemidiaphragm by gas in the left colon.

The junction of the diaphragm with the thoracic wall is termed the *costo-phrenic angle* or *sulcus.* The junction of the diaphragm with the heart silhouette is termed the *cardiophrenic angle.* Normally the costophrenic angles are acute and radiolucent. On some occasions, for example in emphysema, the diaphragms may be so low as to obliterate the costophrenic angles, with no other pathology demonstrated. The cardiophrenic angles are also acute and radiolucent, but it is common to see them obscured by fat depositions.

The diaphragm is best evaluated by means of fluoroscopic procedures, during which the patient can be rotated and the entire diaphragm evaluated. As mentioned previously, it is better to evaluate the diaphragm in both the upright and the recumbent positions, since there is a vast difference in movement of the diaphragm between the two positions.

Mediastinum

The mediastinum is the space containing the heart, great blood vessels, trachea, esophagus, and lymphoid tissue; and it separates the two lungs. It extends from the thoracic inlet and is bounded by the thoracic spine and first ribs superiorly and the diaphragm inferiorly, and from the sternum anteriorly to the thoracic spine posteriorly.

Four arbitrary divisions of the mediastinum are noted; however, in actual roentgenographic practice only three divisions are used. The anatomical superior mediastinum is defined as that portion of the mediastinum superior to a trans-verse plane between the angle of Louis and the inferior portion of T-4. In actual practice, many radiologists would prefer to divide the mediastinum into three approximately equal areas — the anterior, middle, and posterior divisions.

The anterior mediastinum is anterior to a coronal plane between the upper portion of the manubrium to the diaphragm below and contains primarily lymphoid tissue and the thyroid and thymus glands. The posterior mediastinum is that portion of the mediastinum which is posterior to a coronal plane drawn from the posterior portion of the trachea to the diaphragm below and contains mostly the thoracic spine, nervous tissue, esophagus, and descending aorta. The middle mediastinum is that portion between the anterior and posterior medias-tinum and contains the heart, pericardium, ascending aorta, major vessels, trachea, carina, major bifurcation of the trachea, roots of the lungs, and lym-phoid tissue.

One may remember the mediastinal divisions by assuming that the front of the cardiac silhouette is anterior, the heart shadow is middle, and the portion behind the heart is posterior. This division of the mediastinum is important since most mass lesions of the mediastinum can be diagnosed simply by knowing the location of the lesion within the mediastinum (Fig. 10-7). For example, a lesion in the anterior mediastinum would most likely arise from the compo-nents of that area; namely the thymus, thyroid, or lymphoid tissue. The same also applies to the posterior mediastinum, for a posterior mass lesion is most likely to arise from neurogenic, bony, aortic, or esophageal tissue. Midmediastinal mass lesions are most commonly of lymphoid tissue or tumors arising from the roots of the lungs.

ROENTGENOGRAPHIC CONSIDERATIONS

Before entering into any further discussion concerning the chest, some important factors relative to the chest roentgenogram must be noted. There is no substitute for quality in chest roentgenography. Changes in position, respiration, exposure factors, and even centering of the x-ray beam may affect anatomical relationships and create difficulty in interpretation of the film. Consistency is also important, since a large portion of chest radiology deals with comparison of one study to another.

First of all, the patient must be straight. The anterior margins of the clavicles should be equidistant from the spinous processes of the thoracic vertebrae. If the patient is rotated, one hilar area will be accentuated and the size of the other decreased. One lung will also appear darker than the other, and the cardiac silhouette will change. However, rotation may be useful in localization of a lesion and in helping to differentiate hilar masses from vascular shadows.

Degree of inspiratory effort is important. Successful inspiration is measured in adults by noting that the hemidiaphragm is at the level of T-11 and in children by being able to recognize six anterior ribs and eight posterior ribs. If the patient does not take a deep breath, the heart is pushed up in a transverse manner and there is crowding of the pulmonary markings in the lower lung fields which may even present the picture of congestive heart failure (Fig. 10-8). Expiratory films are also helpful. In some patients, expiratory films may be used to evaluate a suspected pneumothorax, since in expiration a pneumothorax appears larger than on inspiration. A double-exposed expiratory and inspiratory film may be used to evaluate movement of the hemidiaphragm (Fig. 10-9).

The film must be properly exposed, and it is generally accepted that one should be able to see the thoracic spine through the cardiac silhouette. If at all possible, the film should be taken at a standard six-foot focal—film distance, since films taken at a shorter focal—film distance magnify organs and shadows do not appear as sharp as when the exposure is made at a longer distance. The angle of the x-ray tube is even important, since the projection of the x-ray beam may cast one shadow upon another and introduce a confusing roentgen anatomy. Portable films are mentioned only to be condemned. Portables should never be used except for examination of patients unable to be brought to the x-ray department.

Occasionally special views are used in chest roentgenography. The Bucky

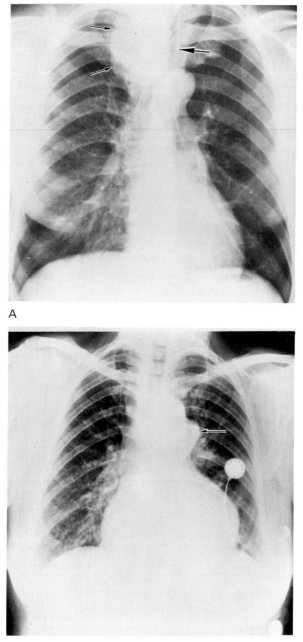

A

B

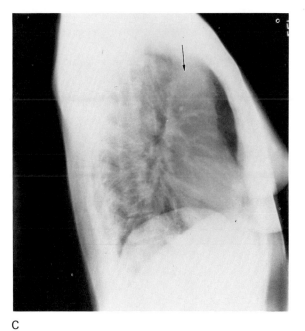

C

Fig. 10-7.

(A) Superior mediastinal mass (substernal thyroid) displacing the trachea (large arrow). (B, C) Posteroanterior and lateral views of a middle mediastinal mass lesion (adenocarcinoma).

film is used to overpenetrate soft tissues and to look for lesions which may be hidden by soft tissue infiltrates. Lateral decubitus films may be used to detect air—fluid levels or pleural fluid. Occasionally a kyphotic or lordotic view is needed to cast the shadows of the clavicle off the upper lung fields for better visualization of the apexes of the lung or the middle lobe. For large patients, a grid may be used to reduce the amount of scattered radiation to the film and hence to lessen fogging of the film by the scattered radiation and present a clearer view of the lung fields.

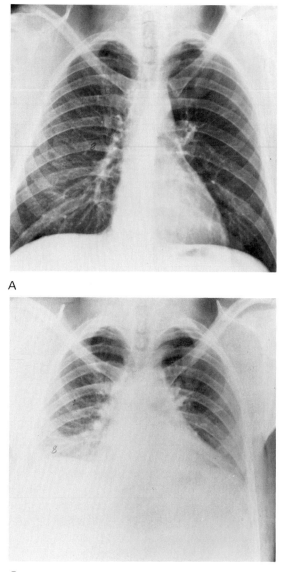

A

B

Fig. 10-8.

(A) Inspiratory chest film. (B) Expiratory film, same patient, with film made only seconds later. Notice how the high diaphragms create an illusion of cardiomegaly.

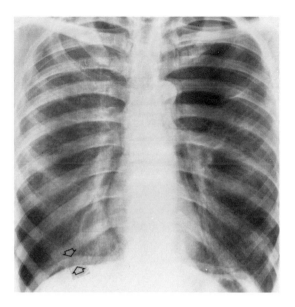

Fig. 10-9.
  Double-exposed inspiratory/expiratory chest film demonstrating diaphragmatic movement.

   Specialized examinations are also used in evaluation of chest lesions. One of the more common procedures is that of tomography (laminography, planigraphy). Tomograms are used to better visualize a lesion. The principle of tomography is that an x-ray film is in a fixed location and is attached by a fulcrum to an x-ray tube so that there is an equidistance at all times between the x-ray tube and the x-ray film. Since there is a relationship between the fulcrum and the focus of the x-ray beam to the film, one has only to move a lesion within the level of focus and all densities above or below this area will be out of focus, or blurred. One is thus able to visualize a particular area without confusing overlying or underlying shadows. The main reasons tomography is used in examination of chest lesions is to delineate calcification within nodules (Fig. 10-10); to evaluate the presence or absence of cavitation within lesions, particularly those located in the apex of the upper lobe or superior segment of the lower lobe; to rule out endobronchial lesions; and to examine the hilar regions for mass lesions. As a general rule, the presence of calcification within a pulmonary nodule would indicate that this is most likely a benign lesion. Lack of calcification in a coin lesion of the lung may be an indication of malignancy.
   One cannot overemphasize the importance of understanding the basic

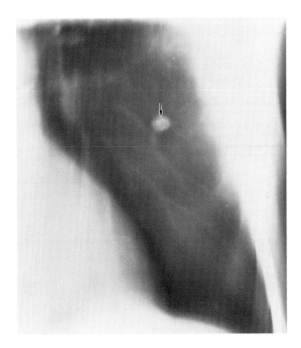

Fig. 10-10.
Tomogram of a nodule in the left lower lobe which demonstrates typical calcification.

principles and anatomy alluded to in the previous paragraphs. Detection of pathological changes within the lungs depends upon the distortion of normal roentgen anatomy as has been presented. As one lecturer [T.T.T.] has so often stated, "God made people in halves so that radiologists can compare one side to another." In reference to the lungs, the radiologist must compare the volume of one lung to that of the other and the density of one part of the lung to the density of a similar portion of the opposite lung.

Changes in lung volume can be secondary to a collapse of a portion of the lung as may result from obstruction to the airway; for example, from a carcinoma, foreign body, or inflammatory reaction. With loss of a portion of the lung volume, the remainder of the lung expands to fill the area. If overexpansion of a lung occurs, the mediastinum may shift toward the opposite side, the ribs may expand to create more thoracic volume, or the diaphragm may be depressed. As lung volume decreases there is elevation of the hemidiaphragm of the affected side, crowding of the ribs, or a movement of the mediastinum toward the affected side.

Loss of lung volume may occur from either intrinsic or extrinsic pathology.

In inflammatory lesions involving the parenchyma of the lung, the resultant scarring or fibrosis may cause loss of volume (atelectasis) with concomitant over-expansion of the adjacent lobes or segments. If a bronchus is compressed from without, there may be inadequate air ingress or egress and resultant poor expansion of the lobe and subsequent resorption of air and loss of volume. In such pathological entities as asthma or emphysema, there may be enlargement of the lung due to overaeration. With changes from either loss of volume or compensatory overinflation, there is a realignment of the bronchi and pulmonary vessels to compensate for the shift in location of the lobes or segments. There is also a resultant shift of the pleural fissures which may also be used to indicate loss or change of volume.

In order to produce a density in the lung, there must be replacement of air sacs with either fluid or tissue. This tissue may be tumor, scarring, fluid, or blood; since all of these have essentially the same roentgen appearance and absorption of radiation, the configuration and location of the density and possibly the duration of the lesion become important. Parenchymal lesions may be spherical or irregular, and generally all margins of the density can be seen. Pleural or extrapleural lesions can also be identified by their configuration (Fig. 10-11). The presence of calcification within the density for example, would

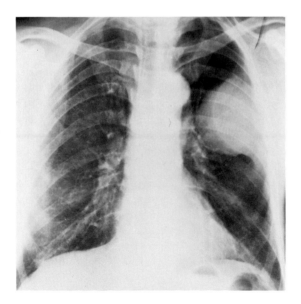

Fig. 10-11.
Typical extrapleural lesion, left lateral chest, demonstrating sharp margins with tapering edges, convexity toward the lung, and rib destruction.

most likely indicate that this is secondary to a previous infection. Cavitation is important.

Therefore to properly evaluate a chest film one must compare the size of one lung to the other, compare the relative radiolucency of one lung to the other, and look for the presence of increased densities, either localized or scattered, throughout the lung field and compare it to a region in the opposite lung field. There is no set pattern that allows one to say, "This is pneumonia," or "This is tumor." The radiologist has developed through experience knowledge of a spectrum of shadows corresponding to various stages of disease processes which allows him to make a valid assumption concerning that disease process.

Pulmonary Emphysema. Unfortunately many authors use the terms *chronic bronchitis* and *emphysema* interchangeably, although the connotation of each is different from that held by our clinical colleagues, pathologists, and radiologists. The two processes are quite commonly associated with one another, and it is unusual to see emphysema that does not have an associated chronic bronchitis. Chronic bronchitis, as the name implies, is a chronic infection of the bronchi. This is demonstrated by bronchography and presents as irregular bronchi with occasional mucus plugging of smaller-ordered bronchioles and dilated mucous glands projecting from the walls of the bronchioles. In those patients having chronic bronchitis, routine films show no roentgen signs unless occasionally one sees a dilated, thickened bronchiole or unless the patient has associated lung changes secondary to his chronic bronchitis.

Pulmonary emphysema is a lung disease characterized by an increase in the air spaces distal to the terminal bronchioles and usually associated with tissue destruction. Chronic bronchitis and emphysema are two of the more commonly seen respiratory tract diseases in a private medical practice. Little can be done to reverse the anatomical changes in emphysema, although a good deal can be done in the management of such a patient. Etiological factors remain uncertain, although cigarette smoking, air pollution, and industrial dust exposure are contributory.

In radiology there are two basic types of emphysema seen, that with air trapping and that without. Emphysema without air trapping, such as compensatory overinflation of the lung following removal of the opposite lung or segment, usually produces no clinical symptoms. Overinflation can be seen roentgenographically only by a change in fissures, shift of the mediastinum, redistribution of the pulmonary vessels or bronchioles, or increased radiolucency of the lung.

Emphysema (Fig. 10-12) with air trapping or, as it is commonly called, chronic obstructive lung disease, is characterized roentgenographically by a flattening of the hemidiaphragms to such a degree as to at least partially obscure the costophrenic angles; an increase in the retrosternal air space; and an irregular hyperlucency of the lung fields. As emphysema progresses, there is diminution of the caliber of the vascular markings in the peripheral lung fields with an associated increase in the hilar shadows. There is a decreased movement of the hemidiaphragms and the AP diameter of the chest increases, sometimes associated with a kyphosis.

As the diaphragms are pushed downward by the entrapped air within the lung, there is elongation of the heart so that the cardiothoracic ratio is out of proportion. The disease process may proceed to such a point that cor pulmonale and right heart failure may occur.

Emphysema may be localized or generalized. Local changes may be suggested by comparing one portion of the lung field with the opposite side. In some patients the localized destruction of the alveoli may be sufficient to produce large emphysematous bullae which are demonstrated roentgenographically as thin-walled, smooth, air-filled blebs. Differentiation of emphysematous bullae from cysts may be difficult. Emphysematous bullae may vary from a few millimeters to several centimeters in diameter (Fig. 10-13).

Carcinoma of the Lung. There are several types of carcinoma of the lung, but usually one speaks of bronchogenic carcinoma and includes such lesions as superior sulcus tumors, adenocarcinomas, lymphoma, and metastatic tumors. Bronchogenic carcinoma is the most common type of tumor seen in the male, with the possible exception of prostatic carcinoma. The overall five-year survival rate is dismal, being only about 12 to 14 percent. Surgical extirpation is the only cure. Unfortunately only approximately half the patients seen at the first visit to the physician are operable.

Etiological factors are unknown, although there is a statistical relationship to cigarette smoking and residence in an industrial area of high air pollution; hence the average patient is a male heavy cigarette smoker living in an urban area and generally over the age of 45. There does appear to be a correlation between the amount of cigarette smoking and the incidence of carcinoma. Those patients smoking less than ten cigarettes a day are at the same risk level as nonsmokers; as the number of cigarettes smoked per day increases, so does the incidence of tumor. To indicate the degree of cigarette smoking by a patient, clinicians have recently referred to *pack-years* — namely, the number of packages of cigarettes smoked daily and for how many years. For example, a patient smoking two packs of cigarettes a day for twenty years would be a forty pack-years person.

Standard PA and lateral chest films are the best screening procedure for bronchogenic carcinoma. Unfortunately, roentgenograms cannot make a tissue diagnosis, but they do serve to direct the clinician toward an etiological factor for a mass within the chest. Cytological studies of sputum and bronchial washings or brushings are the most conservative diagnostic procedures short of surgical biopsy. Unless the tumor connects directly to a bronchus and there is movement of sputum from the area of the tumor through the trachea, cytological studies will be negative.

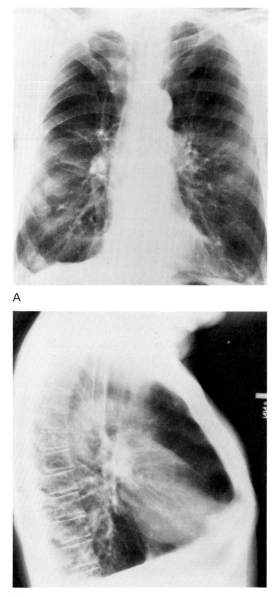

A

B

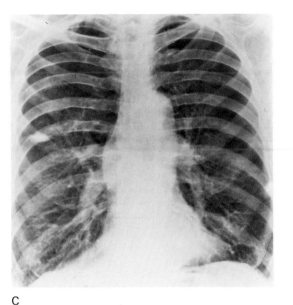

C

Fig. 10-12.

Pulmonary emphysema. (A, B) Notice the flat hemidiaphragms, increased retrosternal air space, and irregular hyperlucency of the lung fields. (C) Emphysema with large blebs in the upper lung fields and chronic lung changes in the lower lung fields. Even though the blebs are not well seen on the reproduction, a marked difference between the penetration (blackness) of the upper lung fields as compared to the lower lung fields is apparent. The density in the right midlung is an old scar.

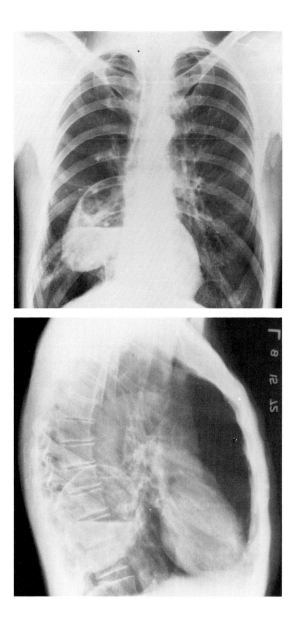

Fig. 10-13.
Multiple bilateral lung cysts, with one partially filled with fluid.

Special roentgenographic procedures such as tomography are helpful to detect calcific deposits within coin lesions, to demonstrate evidence of an endobronchial mass lesion, or to show sources of extrinsic pressure on the bronchus (Fig. 10-14). During the past few years bronchography with concomitant scraping of the suspected bronchus have added to the diagnostic armamentarium of radiologists.

Carcinoma of the lung can have so many frank and subtle forms that the radiologist must always be careful that insidious changes are not cast off in favor of some inconsequential pulmonary lesion. In looking at a number of cases of bronchogenic carcinoma a few years ago, the most common roentgenographic presentation was that of a perihilar mass, which occurs in about one-third of the cases. Solitary lung nodules, or coin lesions, as they are commonly referred to, were the second most common presentation. A collapsed or atelectatic segment, slowly resolving or recurring localized pneumonitis, cavitating lesions, and pleural effusions were the presenting roentgen signs in the majority of the other cases. The presence of pleural effusion, mediastinal adenopathy, and pleural implants usually indicates that the tumor is far advanced and not surgically removable. Perihilar masses are usually associated with symptoms of cough and, occasionally, pain. Solitary nodules are usually found on chest films taken for other reasons; for example, hospital admission chest films or screening films for tuberculosis.

One cannot overemphasize that in order for a cure to be obtained in carcinoma of the lung, early detection is mandatory. To reiterate, minimal signs or symptoms of pulmonary disease should be examined roentgenographically with at least a chest film. High-risk male patients of age 45 or over residing in a high air-pollution area should have periodic chest films to screen for early curable bronchogenic carcinoma. Figures 10-15 through 10-20 are typical examples of lung cancers.

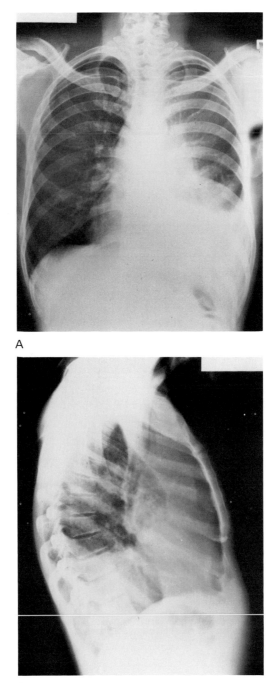

A

B

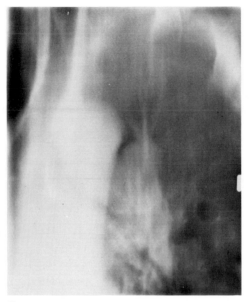

C

Fig. 10-14.
(A—C) Bronchogenic carcinoma of the left lower lobe, with an associated pleural effusion. Tomogram shows a large left hilar mass (C). Compare the hilum with that in Figures 10-5A, B.

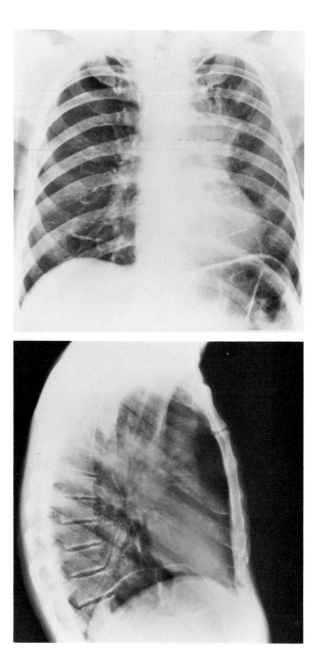

Fig. 10-15.
Oat cell carcinoma, left hilum.

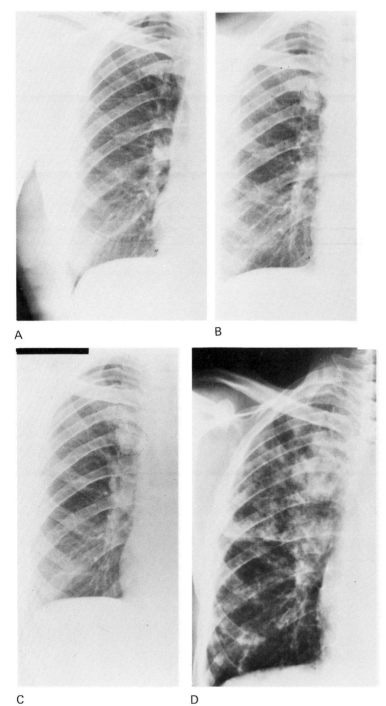

A   B

C   D

Fig. 10-16.
(A–D) Development of a bronchogenic carcinoma over a two-year period.

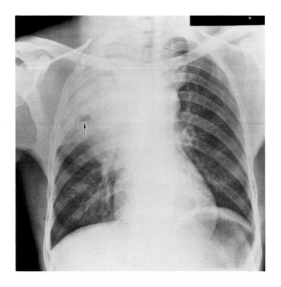

Fig. 10-17.
Carcinoma of the right upper lobe, with associated lung abscess.

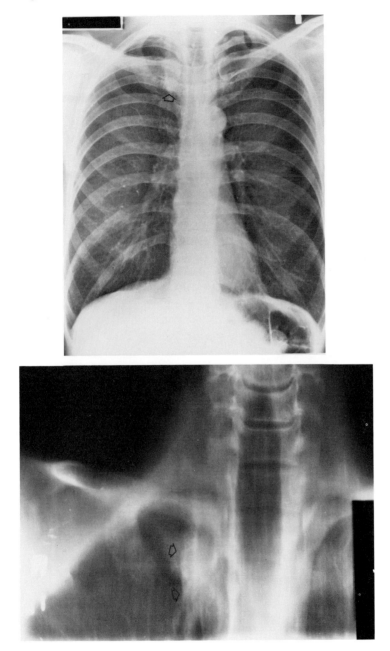

Fig. 10-18.
 Carcinoma of the right upper lobe, better demonstrated with a tomogram. The tumor is magnified on the tomogram (bottom).

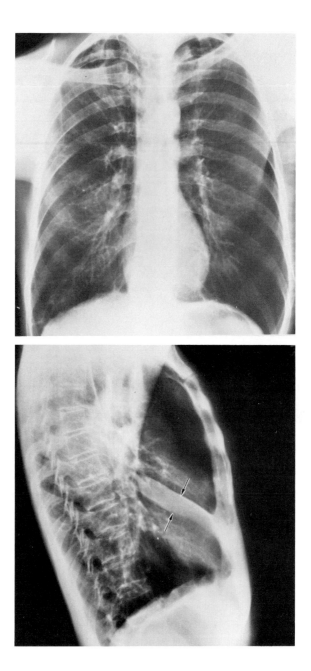

Fig. 10-19.
  Right middle lobe atelectasis due to endobronchial tumor. Notice how the collapse is better seen on the lateral film.

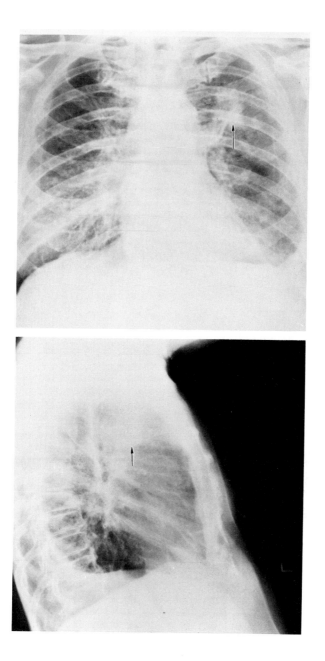

Fig. 10-20.

Bronchogenic carcinoma, anterior segment, left upper lobe, with pleural effusion. Notice the congested vessels in the right lower lobe.

Tuberculosis. Only a few decades ago tuberculosis was the leading cause of death in this country. Following pasteurization of milk, bovine tuberculosis has become exceedingly rare, so that today almost all tuberculosis seen is that caused by the human bacillus and the primary infection is pulmonary in nature.

Primary tuberculosis is seldom seen in adults and is limited mostly to infants and children. In the young, primary tuberculosis consists of a peripheral infiltrate located generally subpleurally and in the lower lung fields. This is combined with enlargement of the hilar and mediastinal lymph nodes. As the lesion heals, calcified lymph nodes remain to attest to the tuberculous infection (Fig. 10-21).

In the adult, tuberculosis is a reinfection; that is to say, the patient has been reinfected with the tubercle bacillus, either from an exogenous source or from dormant bacilli remaining from a previous infection. The site of infection is more frequently in the apical segment of the upper lobes or in the superior segments of the lower lobe. The infiltrate may expand, involving the entire segments of the lobe, and may produce cavitation (Fig. 10-22). The cavity may break through the bronchus and spread the bacilli throughout the lung, producing bronchogenic tuberculosis (Fig. 10-23). Spread by vascular routes produces miliary tuberculosis (Fig. 10-24). At any time and with proper therapy, the tuberculosis process may be controlled and the disease regressed. Pleural effusion and involvement of the pericardium may also be seen and, with resultant healing, produce calcification of the pleura and pericardium (Fig. 10-25). In the adult, lymph node enlargement in response to tuberculosis is unusual. As initially seen on the roentgenogram, tuberculosis appears as bilateral upper lobe infiltrates, either with or without cavitation or marked pleural reaction. If the same type of infiltrate appears only in segments other than the apical or superior portions, doubt should be raised as to whether the diagnosis of tuberculosis is correct.

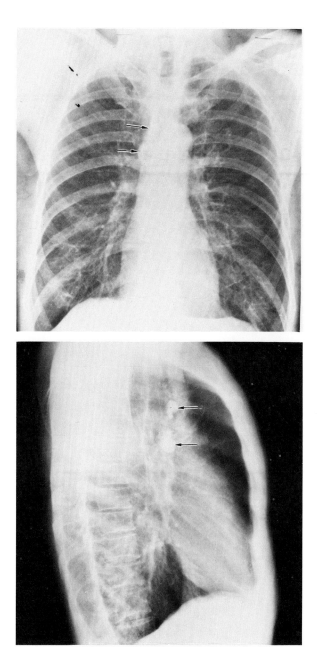

Fig. 10-21.
Calcified paratracheal lymph nodes from previous tuberculosis.

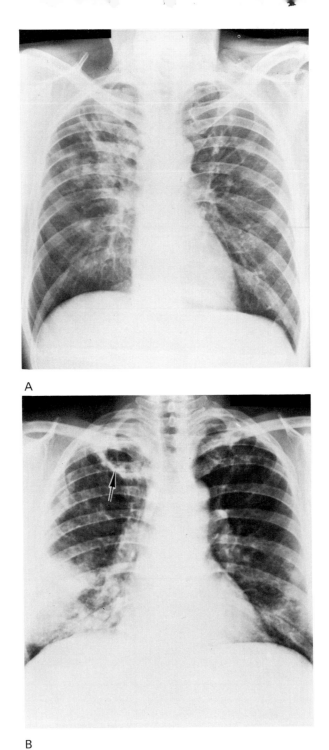

A

B

Fig. 10-22.

Active tuberculosis. (A) The average case of tuberculosis presents with bilateral apical infiltrates similar to those seen in this patient. Tomograms demonstrated cavitation in the right upper lobe. (B) Large, obvious cavity in the right upper lobe with bronchogenic spread to lower lobes.

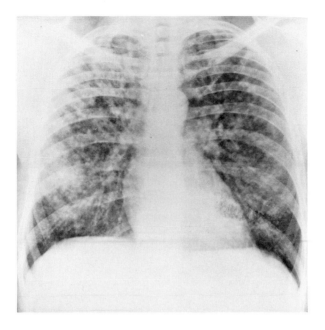

Fig. 10-23.
Marked bronchogenic spread of tuberculosis. Notice that the lesions vary in size.

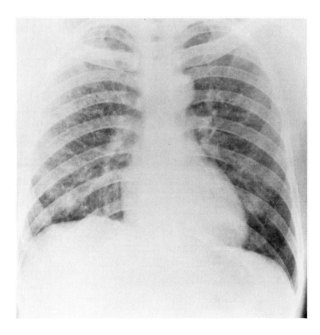

Fig. 10-24.
Miliary tuberculosis. Notice how small and uniform the lesions are, and compare to those in Figure 10-23.

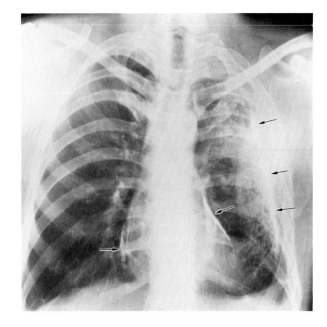

Fig. 10-25.
Marked pleural and pericardial calcification from tuberculosis.

Pneumonia. The terms *pneumonia* and *pneumonitis* are used interchangeably. Pneumonia by strict definition is inflammation of the lungs associated with clinical symptoms, and pneumonitis is a localized pneumonia that produces no clinical reaction. Lobar pneumonia involves the entire segment of lung, and bronchopneumonia commonly refers to patchy pneumonic processes which may coalesce and produce consolidation.

Pneumococcal pneumonia is the type more commonly seen in the physician's office. The pneumonia generally is preceded by an upper respiratory infection and is subsequently followed by chills, cough, chest pain, and high fever. Roentgenographic findings may be less pronounced than physical findings but may show lobar consolidation (Fig. 10-26).

In hospitals one more commonly sees pneumonia secondary to gram-negative or staphylococcal infections. These pneumonias generally occur secondary to other disease entities such as influenza, malignancy, human organ transplantations, and so on. Pneumatoceles are commonly associated with staphylococcal pneumonia. *Klebsiella* pneumonia may be suspected from its rapid spreading course and swift development of pulmonary abscesses.

Viral pneumonias appear more commonly than a few years ago and usually occur in small epidemic outbreaks. Onset is vague, and the patient may complain

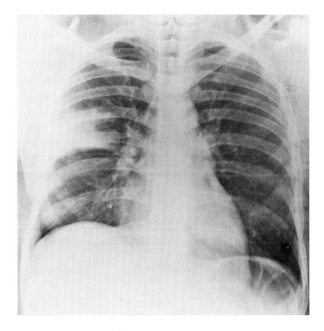

Fig. 10-26.
Pneumococcal pneumonia, anterior segment, right upper lobe.

of flulike symptoms. Roentgenographic findings are usually much more pronounced than the physical findings would indicate.

Aspiration pneumonia is frequently seen, particularly in hospitals. The pneumonia occurs as a result of aspiration of foreign material (usually gastric contents) into the lungs (Fig. 10-27). It occurs most often in postoperative patients and in alcoholics due to the loss of the cough reflex. The presence of the aspirated foreign material irritates the air passages and produces edema, which serves as an excellent culture site for pathological bacteria.

Aspiration pneumonia may be suspected from the localization of the pneumonic process. These infiltrations are located posteriorly in the lower part of the upper lobes or in the superior segments of the lower lobes. The appearance of aspiration pneumonia in other lobes is unusual.

The presence of a pneumonic process initially blurs lung markings, and one sees on the roentgenogram widening of the vascular shadows which are somewhat blurred in comparison to other areas within the lung fields. As the edema created by the pneumonia progresses, the interstitial tissues surrounding the bronchi become engorged with fluid, so that one may see small bronchioles containing air. This appearance has been termed the *air-bronchogram sign,* which was popularized by Dr. Benjamin Felson. Fluid-filled alveoli progressively

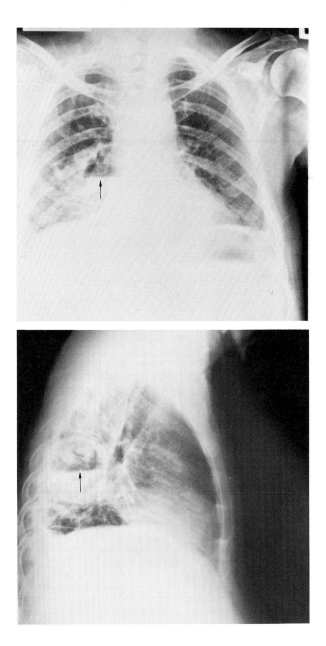

Fig. 10-27.
Aspiration pneumonia with abscess, superior segment, right lower lobe.

coalesce so that irregular, fluffy densities are seen on the roentgenogram. These densities may be localized or scattered throughout the lung fields. In viral pneumonias the infiltrates are perihilar in location, producing a butterfly-shaped distribution of the infiltrate. On some occasions differentiation between pulmonary edema secondary to heart or renal failure and inflammatory exudates may be difficult; and one may have to rely upon a clinical evaluation of the patient to make a diagnosis.

Lung Abscesses and Empyema. A lung abscess is a localized necrosis of pulmonary tissue surrounded by inflammatory debris. Abscesses are most commonly due to obstruction of a bronchus by tumor, mucus plugs, blood, and the debris from pneumonic processes. Septic emboli, cavitating cancers, and infarction also may produce changes consistent with lung abscesses.

Signs and symptoms of lung abscesses are those of pneumonia, and there is subsequent expectoration of large volumes of infected sputum.

Roentgenographically, an abscess demonstrates an air—fluid level within a cavity. Surrounding the cavity is usually a large, thick-walled capsule. Pleural effusion may also be present. Fluid-filled cysts may give the same appearance, but usually the wall is thinner (see Fig. 10-13).

At times it may be difficult to differentiate a peripheral lung abscess from empyema. Empyemas (Fig. 10-28) are purulent exudates in the pleural cavity occurring as a complication or extension of an inflammatory reaction elsewhere in the chest. Empyemas may also result from penetrating chest wounds or from surgical intervention within the thorax. Generally, the appearance is that of a free or localized pleural effusion; but air—fluid levels are commonly seen. Differentiation between empyemas and lung abscesses is important, since the abscesses are treated initially with expectorants, antibiotics, and postural drainage. Insertion of a chest tube into the pleural space and heavy antibiotic therapy are the normal initial treatments for empyema.

One should realize that the most common etiology of both empyema and abscess is obstruction of bronchi, either intrinsically or extrinsically. Hence, routine tomographic examination of the bronchi should be obtained, followed by bronchography if indicated. A rather marked inflammatory reaction about an abscess may obscure bronchial obstruction, and it is generally better to wait for one to two weeks after initiation of medical therapy before performing tomography.

Lung abscesses and empyemas may resolve completely, leaving a small amount of scar tissue residue (Fig. 10-29). If cavitation from the lung abscess is sufficient, there will be loss of volume of that particular segment of the lung, with resultant changes in elevation of the hemidiaphragm and movement of the hilar vessels to compensate for the loss in chest volume. A late complication of either an abscess or an empyema is a bronchopleural fistula in which there is consistent recontamination of the abscess and empyema via bacteria flowing through the fistula.

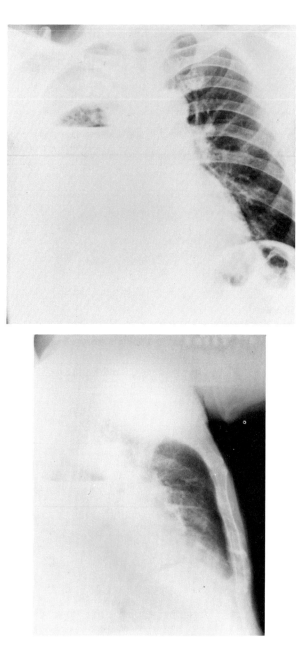

Fig. 10-28.

Marked opacification of the right chest from empyema. Notice the air—fluid level. This patient subsequently developed a bronchopleural fistula.

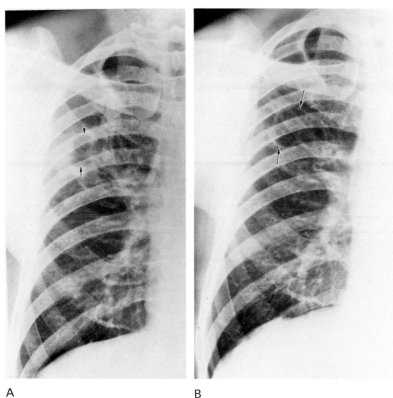

A   B

Fig. 10-29.

(A) Abscess, right upper lobe. (B) Months later, a cyst remains in place of the abscess.

Sarcoidosis. Sarcoidosis was selected for presentation in this text because of its protean manifestations in the lung. Hilar or mediastinal adenopathy, interstitial nodularity, chronic fibrotic changes, cystic emphysema, or a combination of each of these may be seen roentgenographically from the disease process. Like syphilis, which has been described in the past as the "great pretender" or "great imitator," sarcoidosis can also mimic a host of disease processes such as miliary tuberculosis, viral pneumonia, lymphoma, carcinoma, or pneumoconiosis.

Unlike tuberculosis or lymphoma, sarcoid nodes are usually hilar in location, well defined, and bilaterally symmetrical. Parenchymal involvement varies from linear interstitial changes to nodularity, with some predilection for the midlung fields. Pleural effusion is extremely rare in sarcoidosis and may be a differential point in diagnosis.

Sarcoidosis is a noncaseating granulomatous disease of unknown etiology. The patient may be asymptomatic or may complain of respiratory distress. Treatment with steroids is common, but there are many patients who spontaneously resolve the disease process without any definitive therapy. However, in some patients the disease may become prolonged and heal with fibrosis and cystic emphysema. Fig. 10-30 shows representative examples of sarcoidosis within the lung.

Pneumothorax. Each lung is encased by serous fibromembrane called the *visceral pleura.* This is continuous with the parietal pleura which lines the inner surface of the thoracic cage, upper surface of the diaphragm, and the lateral surface of the mediastinum. A potential space is present between the two sheets of pleura; but unless some pathological process separates the pleurae, this space cannot be detected roentgenographically.

Admission of free air into the pleural space results in a pneumothorax and collapse of the lung. Pneumothoraxes may be secondary to trauma or may occur spontaneously. Traumatic pneumothoraxes result from penetration of the thorax by wounds, crushing trauma, or any force in which air may be admitted to the pleural cavity. Pneumothoraxes may also result from thoracentesis in which a bronchus is inadvertently punctured during the procedure (Fig. 10-31). Spontaneous pneumothoraxes may result from some pulmonary disease processes such as emphysema, tuberculosis, carcinoma, or spontaneous rupture of peripheral blebs, as well as severe coughing spells.

Signs and symptoms of pneumothorax are related to the degree of pneumothorax. Usually there is a history of acute onset of sharp chest pain associated with a nonproductive cough and shortness of breath. As the pressure in the chest equalizes, symptoms may abate.

Roentgenographically, pneumothorax is characterized by absence of peripheral lung markings. In most cases the visceral pleura may be readily visualized. Tension pneumothoraxes occur as a result of ingress of air into the pleural cavity with egress prohibited because of a ball-valve mechanism; and with every

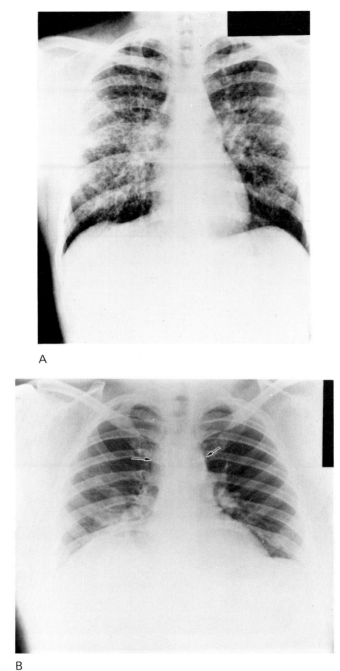

A

B

Figure 10-30.
(Legend on page 261.)

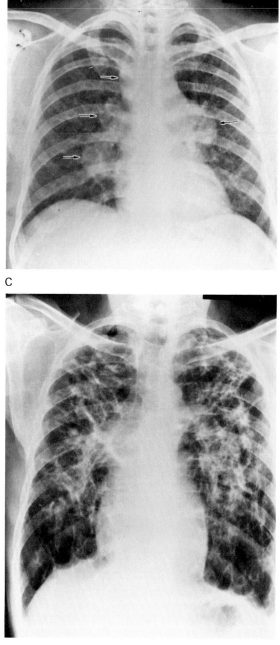

C

D

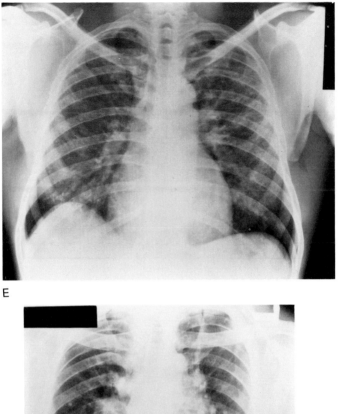

E

F

Fig. 10-30.

The many faces of sarcoidosis. Each presentation is different and resembles another pathological entity such as: (A) pneumoconiosis, (B) mediastinal tumor, (C) lymphoma, (D) chronic lung disease with emphysema, (E) bronchogenic tuberculosis, (F) carcinoma.

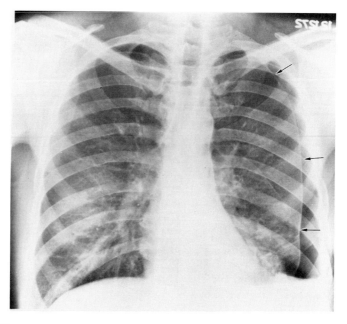

Fig. 10-31.

   Left pneumothorax secondary to diagnostic thoracentesis. Notice the carcinoma in the left hilum.

breath the pressure in the pleural cavity increases. This increasing pressure shifts the mediastinum and compromises circulation (Fig. 10-32). An effective emergency treatment of a tension pneumothorax is to insert a large needle into the pneumothorax so that the intrapleural and extrapleural pressures can be equalized.

On some occasions history may be suggestive of a pneumothorax but none is found roentgenographically. In these cases an expiratory chest film will provide an enlarged view of the pneumothorax. Sometimes adhesions in the pleural space may prevent collapse of the lung, and one may see a localized pneumothorax.

Pleural effusions often result from inflammatory or carcinomatous disease of the lung parenchyma and are almost invariably associated with prolonged congestive heart failure (Fig. 10-33). Small amounts of effusion (less than 100 ml) are not usually detected roentgenographically. When such effusions are present, the costophrenic sulci are rounded and the diaphragms may be elevated. Since scar tissue may also blunt the costophrenic angles, a lateral decubitus film should be obtained before proceeding with a pleural tap for diagnosis (Fig. 10-34).

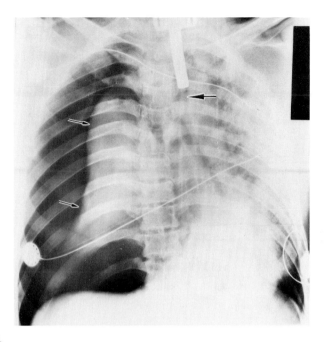

Fig. 10-32.
Tension pneumothorax with almost complete collapse of the right lung and with the mediastinum shifted to the left. The patient is rotated slightly to the left.

The preceding discussion concerning the lung and mediastinum covers the vast majority of conditions seen in the chest. This is not to say that such entities as collagen diseases, pneumoconiosis, pulmonary emboli, or chronic interstitial fibrosis are not just as important. By recognizing the abnormalities that have been presented, the student will better appreciate the less common diseases seen in the thorax.

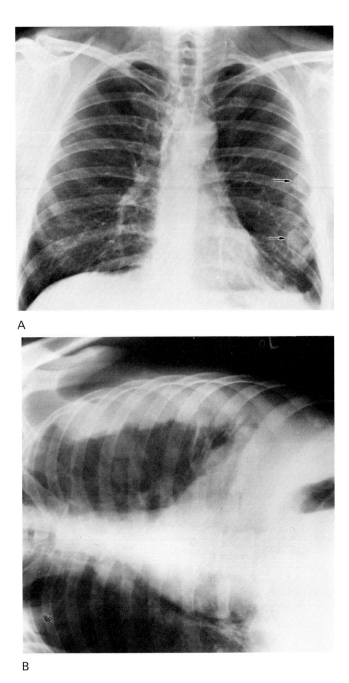

A

B

Fig. 10-33.

(A) Pleural plaques remaining from old infection. Compare to Figure 10-11.
(B) Lateral decubitus film demonstrating multiple metastatic pleural lesions. Parenchymal nodules are also seen.

264

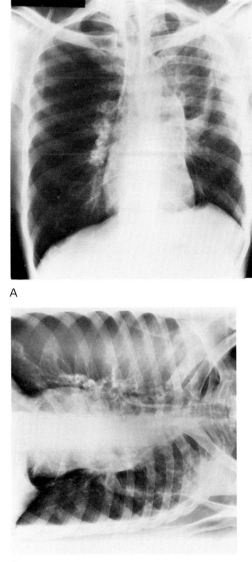

A

B

Fig. 10-34.
 Subpulmonic effusion. (A) Carcinoma of the left hilum with apparently clear costophrenic angles. The left hemidiaphragm is elevated. (B) Same patient; left lateral decubitus
film showing pleural effusion. Notice the linear density extending from the left hilum.
This is not an abscess since the air—fluid level does not change on the decubitus film.

READING LIST

Felson, B. *Fundamentals of Chest Roentgenology.* Philadelphia: Saunders, 1960.
Felson, B., Weinstein, A. S., and Spitz, H. B. *Principles of Chest Roentgenology.* Philadelphia: Saunders, 1965.
Fraser, R. G., and Paré, J. A. P. *Diagnosis of Diseases of the Chest.* Philadelphia: Saunders, 1970.
Hinshaw, H. C., and Garland, L. H. *Diseases of the Chest.* Philadelphia: Saunders, 1963.
Simon, G. *Principles of Chest X-Ray Diagnosis.* London: Butterworth, 1962.

The Heart and Great Vessels 11

THE HEART is a tubular structure occupying the major portion of the mediastinum in the normal person. It is composed of four chambers — two ventricles and two atria. The right atrium receives unoxygenated blood from the systemic circulation through the superior and inferior vena cavae. It empties through the tricuspid valve into the right ventricle. The right ventricle acts as a pump to force unoxygenated blood through the pulmonic valve and into the pulmonary artery. About 60 percent of the blood flow is to the right lung and capillary bed, with the remainder permeating the left pulmonary vascular system. Through a complicated system of pressures, resistances, flow, and exchange mechanisms, the blood is oxygenated in the capillary bed and flows back through the pulmonary veins into the left atrium and through the mitral valve to the left ventricle. The left ventricle is more muscular than the right ventricle and pumps oxygenated blood at systemic pressures through the aortic valve. The aortic arch exits anterosuperiorly from the left ventricle and courses superiorly and laterally, giving off the innominate artery (which branches into the right subclavian, carotid, and vertebral arteries), left subclavian artery, and left vertebral artery before descending posteroinferiorly.

ROENTGENOGRAPHIC CONSIDERATIONS

The standard roentgenogram of the heart is taken with the patient in the PA position with the focal—film distance a minimum of six feet (two meters) to decrease the magnification of the heart. Films taken at this distance allow approximately a 10 percent magnification factor which would be increased if the focal—film distance were less. If the film were taken in the AP rather than the PA projection, a small increase in magnification would be present because the heart is an anterior structure. If the inspiratory effort is not as full as it

should be, the high diaphragms may create a transverse appearance to the heart
and cause a false engorgement of the pulmonary vessels, particularly in the lower
lung fields, thus presenting a picture compatible with congestive heart failure.
In this regard one should evaluate the level of the diaphragms, which should be
at approximately the T-11 level before considering a full inspiratory effort to be
present. A full inspiration obviously is difficult to obtain in patients who are
obese or in those who have thoracic or spinal abnormalities or who may have
concomitant thoracic or abdominal pain in which the pain reflex prevents full
inspiration. Patients should not be rotated; thus there should be an equal distance of the ends of the clavicles from the spinous processes of the thoracic
spine. Even a slight degree of rotation on the PA film may accentuate the heart
and hilar areas, creating a false impression of cardiac enlargement.

The presence of a pectus excavatum should be evaluated with a lateral film,
as a pectus may decrease the AP diameter of the chest, forcing the heart into a
smaller area and creating the appearance of cardiac enlargement on the AP or
PA film with the shift of the heart to the left. The presence of a pectus cari-
natum generally will not affect the cardiac size. The cardiac silhouette may be
shifted to one side or the other secondary to disease processes elsewhere in the
chest, for example, scarring of a lung field secondary to tuberculosis and pulling
of the mediastinum to the side of disease. A tension pneumothorax may shift
the cardiac silhouette to the opposite side of its normal location. The presence
of severe pulmonary emphysema may depress the diaphragm to an abnormal
level and at the same time elongate the heart, creating the appearance of a
smaller cardiac silhouette than one would expect if the diaphragms were at the
normal level. Another factor to consider in the evaluation of the heart size is
the degree of engorgement of the pulmonary and systemic blood systems. In
severe dehydration the blood volume is decreased and there may be a concomitant decrease in cardiac size; or conversely the patient may be overhydrated
with an increased cardiac blood pool, creating an enlargement of the cardiac
silhouette. The presence of a significant pericardial effusion may create an
enlargement of the cardiac silhouette without a concomitant increase in the
cardiac size.

All the above factors must be appreciated by the radiologist before he attempts
to evaluate cardiac size or shape. If one does not evaluate these factors, a false
impression of cardiac pathology may be determined when the changes actually
are secondary to other factors and not necessarily related to cardiac pathology.
One should also remember that there is a systolic and a diastolic movement of
the heart and that the average change of heart size from the systolic to the
diastolic phase is 1 to 1.5 cm. If, for example, a chest roentgenogram is taken
with the patient in the systolic cardiac cycle, the heart may appear smaller than
if the film were taken a second later when the cardiac cycle is in the diastolic
phase. It has been shown that cardiac motion may in itself increase the cardiac
silhouette, and in this regard it has been suggested that cardiac films be taken
at no less than a 1/10-second exposure time.

In this modern age of medicine one should also consider that there are other means of evaluating cardiac performance in addition to the radiological methods. The introduction of cardiac catheterization and recording of pressures within each individual chamber and dye curve analysis are fully needed in proper evaluation of cardiac performance or pathology.

The Cardiac Series. The basic tool of evaluation of cardiac performance and pathology is the cardiac series, which is a study done in conjunction with fluoroscopy of the heart. The cardiac series is obtained with the patient in four basic positions, namely, the PA, the LAO (left anterior oblique) at 60 degrees, the RAO (right anterior oblique) at 45 degrees, and the true lateral. Since it is difficult to achieve these positions, knowledge that the degree of rotation may vary from examination to examination should be taken into consideration by the radiologist when interpreting the study.

On the PA film (Fig. 11-1) the right heart border is composed primarily of the right atrium. The right pulmonary trunk lies just above the right atrial silhouette. On the left side the pulmonary trunk presents as a straight or slightly concave vascular structure inferior and medial to the aortic knob. Just below the pulmonary trunk the left atrial appendage may be noted. The lower left cardiac border is composed of the left ventricle. The right ventricle occupies the midportion of the cardiac silhouette. The right heart border projects slightly to the right of the thoracic spine, and the apex of the heart intermingles with the left hemidiaphragm. There is generally no projection of the left ventricle (apex of the heart) below the level of the diaphragm.

In the LAO projection (Fig. 11-2) the anterior cardiac silhouette is composed of the right ventricle inferiorly and the right atrial appendage superiorly. However, under normal conditions the anterior border is almost always formed by the right ventricle alone. The posterior cardiac silhouette is composed inferiorly by the left ventricle, which may project slightly over the thoracic spine. Just above the level of the left ventricle is the region of the left atrium. Superior to the left atrium is the so-called pulmonary window, composed superiorly by the left main-stem bronchus and superomedially by the carina and pulmonary great vessels. Left atrial enlargement usually causes an opacity encroaching upon the pulmonary window superiorly and posteriorly. Coursing posteriorly from the level of the carina, the left pulmonary artery can be seen as it enters the left lung. One may also see the aorta emerging from the anterior cardiac silhouette on the LAO view as it curves superoposteriorly, giving off the great vessels to the heart and neck and the vessels for the upper extremities.

The RAO position (Fig. 11-3) shows the apex of the heart pointing toward the left costophrenic angle, and in this position one may see a good portion of the right ventricular outflow tract. The anteroinferior edge of the cardiac silhouette is composed of the left ventricle. The left portion of the silhouette comprises the left atrium superiorly and the right atrium inferiorly.

On the lateral projection (Fig. 11-4) the anterior part of the cardiac silhouette

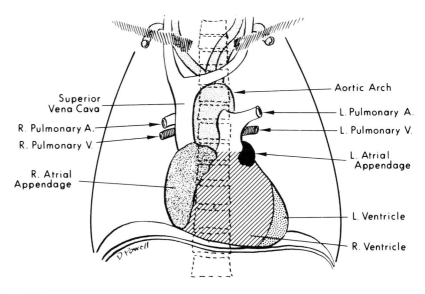

Fig. 11-1.

Anatomical landmarks of the heart, posteroanterior projection.

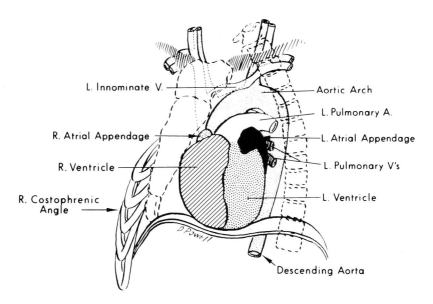

Fig. 11-2.

Anatomical landmarks of the heart, left anterior oblique projection.

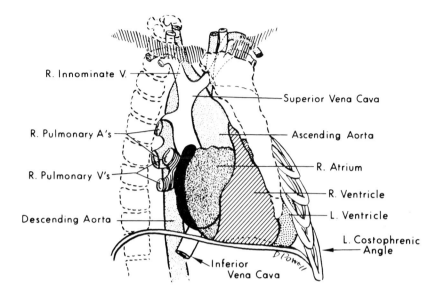

Fig. 11-3.
Anatomical landmarks of the heart, right anterior oblique projection.

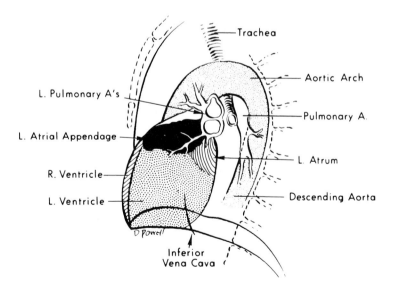

Fig. 11-4.
Anatomical landmarks of the heart, left lateral projection.

is composed of the right ventricle, with the posterior cardiac silhouette composed inferiorly by the left ventricle, which is superimposed upon the inferior vena cava, and superiorly by the left atrium.

In performing a roentgenographic cardiac series the above projections are evaluated against a barium-filled esophagus to better outline the position of the esophagus in reference to the particular chambers of the heart. The esophagus is filled in all views except the LAO, since barium in the esophagus on this partic- ular view may obliterate the pulmonary window and prevent appreciation of subtle changes in the left atrial appendage. At the same time the cardiac series is performed, fluoroscopy is obtained in order to evaluate the pulsations of the pulmonary vessels, to appreciate any significant or subtle enlargement of an individual chamber, or to detect calcification. Figure 11-5 is a normal cardiac series.

In children the cardiac size is difficult to evaluate, and one must depend upon the degree of pulmonary vascularity and the contour of the cardiac silhouette to detect cardiac abnormalities. The x-ray picture of pulmonary vascularity coupled with the contour of the cardiac silhouette, electrocardiogram, and auscultatory findings is very effective in evaluating the pediatric heart. Pediatric cardiac eval- uation is beyond the scope of this presentation, and we shall limit our discussion to the adult heart.

There are many factors which affect cardiac size and must be taken into account when examining a chest film. The major factors are:

1. Degree of respiration or respiratory effort
2. Posture
3. Abnormalities of the thoracic cage
4. Rotation
5. Magnification
6. Degree of the blood vascular volume

Demonstrating Cardiac Enlargement. On the PA film enlargement of the right ventricle may be noted because of a more complete rounding of the cardiac silhouette, particularly toward the apex, and a lifting of the apex off the dia- phragm. Enlargement of the right atrium may cause the right silhouette to project more to the right of the thoracic spine than is normally seen. Left atrial enlargement is seen by an excessive enlargement of the region of the left atrial appendage just below the pulmonary artery. Minor enlargement of the atrial appendage may cause a slight bulge below the pulmonary hilus and in some instances straighten the left heart border. When the left atrium enlarges suffi- ciently, a double density may be seen in the right half of the heart silhouette and may even form a portion of the right cardiac border. As the enlargement increases, the left main-stem bronchus may be elevated, giving another secon- dary sign of left atrial enlargement. Left ventricular enlargement may not be noticed on the PA film, or it may seem that the apex of the heart projects below the level of the hemidiaphragm.

On the LAO view right ventricular enlargement is noted by accentuation of the curve of the anterior cardiac silhouette. Left ventricular enlargement is identified by posteroinferior protrusion of the left ventricular silhouette across the thoracic spine. Enlargement of the left atrium on the LAO view may be noticed by encroachment upon the region of the pulmonary window with accentuation of the cardiac curve in this area and deformity of the barium column.

In the RAO view enlargement of the right and left atrium may be noted by displacement of the barium-filled esophagus. If the enlargement is in the region of the left atrium, the region of the esophagus below the carina will be displaced posteriorly and laterally; and if the right atrium is enlarged, it will be noted more adjacent to the hemidiaphragm. Only severe right atrial enlargement affects the esophagus to any noticeable degree of displacement. Enlargement of the left ventricle may be noted by a projection of the apex of the heart more toward the costrophrenic angle than is normally seen. The enlargement of the pulmonary artery may also be noted in this projection.

On the lateral view, enlargement of the right ventricle may show encroachment upon the retrosternal air space. Enlargement of the left atrium shows displacement of the barium-filled esophagus just below the carina. A valuable indication of left ventricular enlargement is its changed relationship with the inferior vena cava. Normally the left ventricular silhouette does not project more posteriorly than 1.7 cm from the inferior vena cava silhouette measured at a level 2 cm above the crossing point of the inferior vena cava and the posterior cardiac border.

Calcifications. Only occasionally may one pick up cardiac calcification on routine roentgenograms, either of the valves or the coronary arteries. It is rather common to see calcification within the aortic arch, particularly in elderly patients. However, at fluoroscopy one may pick up about 70 percent of calcifications involving the aortic or mitral valve and about one-half the calcifications seen in the coronary arteries. In this regard, if one suspects coronary artery disease or rheumatic heart disease, one should obtain fluoroscopy of the heart to look for calcification. Small calcifications are not seen because of the movement of calcium, blurring out the image on the roentgenogram. Larger calcifications of the valves may be demonstrated by planigraphy.

The preceding anatomical and physiological discussion is by necessity limited to only a small facet of the physiology and anatomy that are known and can be demonstrated by cardiac catheterization and roentgenographic examination. In the forthcoming paragraphs we shall discuss some of the common entities affecting the adult heart which may also be applied to the pediatric patient.

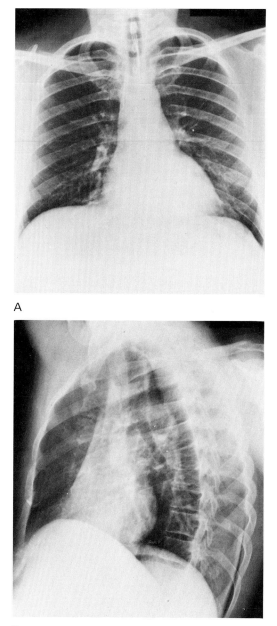

A

B

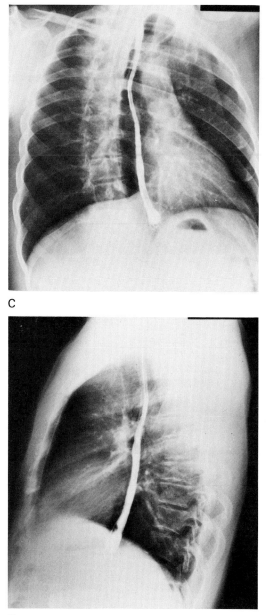

C

D

Fig. 11-5.

(A–D) Normal cardiac series. (A) Posteroanterior view. (B) Left anterior oblique view. (C) Right anterior oblique view. (D) Lateral view. Compare with Figures 11-1 through 11-4.

HEART DISEASE

Rheumatic Heart Disease. This disease is a sequel of infection with beta-hemolytic streptococcus, producing rheumatic fever. A component of rheumatic fever is pancarditis or myocarditis, which may be classified either as active or inactive, and occasionally both forms occur at the same time. Pancarditis may present as congestive heart failure with murmurs and signs of pericarditis. Clinical changes may not be present in sufficient degree to be seen roentgenographically; and, indeed, the patient may have subclinical carditis only to develop clinically significant changes at a later age. The presence of congestive heart failure and cardiac enlargement seen roentgenographically indicate a severe carditis and have an unfavorable prognosis, particularly for the youngster. Carditis in the adult may be of a benign course and clinically insignificant.

The clinically inactive type of rheumatic heart disease is highlighted by endocardial or myocardial damage to some degree. Endocardial damage often occurs at the mitral valve area and occasionally involves the aortic valve. Insufficiency of the valve is more common than stenosis, although both insufficiency and stenosis may occur at the same time. Degrees of severity range from subclinical to marked cardiac disability from valvular or myocardial disease.

Stenosis (Fig. 11-6) is usually due to scarring or adhesions of a portion of one valve leaflet (cusp) to another so as to partially occlude the lumen of the cardiac orifice. Insufficiency is also due to valvular scarring from endocarditis with resultant perforation of the leaflet or curling of the edges of the valve cusp (or leaflet) so that there is no prohibition of the retrograde flow of blood. (In common usage, *insufficiency* is synonymous with *incompetency,* but strictly interpreted *insufficiency* is leakage due to valve deformity whereas *incompetency* relates to a normal-appearing valve leaflet or cusp which does not completely close the cardiac orifice.)

Valvular disease results in altered pressures in adjacent cardiac chambers. One may surmise anticipated changes from the normal blood flow through the heart. As an example, if the mitral valve is partially stenosed, a sufficient amount of blood may not be able to pass through the valve from the left atrium into the left ventricle. The heart has a capability to compensate for this type of damage by simply increasing its rate so that the tissue perfusion with metabolites is maintained at a normal level. As the valve becomes more compromised, the left ventricle cannot supply a sufficient amount of metabolites for tissue needs. At the same time the pressure in the left atrium increases, causing chamber enlargement; the increased pressure within the chamber reflects back through the pulmonary artery and vein to cause changes in the pulmonary vascular bed. As the pressure in the lower pulmonary vasculature increases, there is a constriction of the lower vessels and a concomitant dilatation of the upper vessels, giving the appearance of that which is seen in congestive heart failure.

In mitral insufficiency (Fig. 11-7) the damaged mitral valve does not prevent

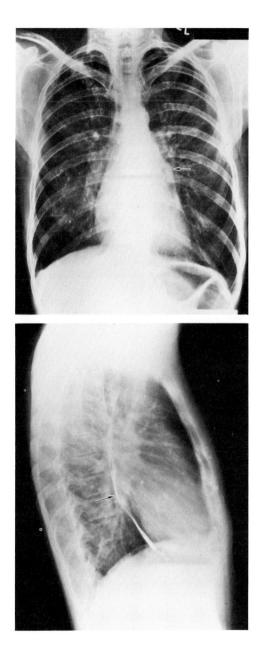

Fig. 11-6.
   Pure mitral valve stenosis. Notice the mild enlargement of the left atrial appendage which straightens the left heart border on the PA view. Typical indentation of the esophageal barium column by left atrial enlargement is noted on the lateral film.

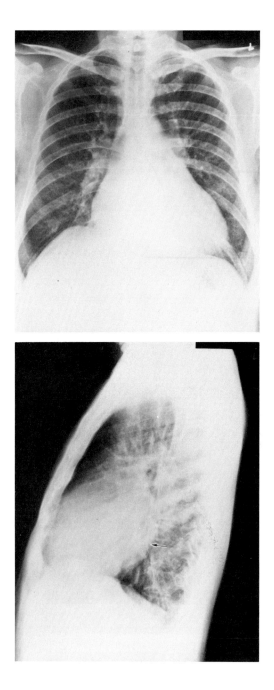

Fig. 11-7.
Pure mitral valve insufficiency. Notice that the heart is larger than is seen in mitral stenosis and that the left atrial enlargement is more prominent.

the retrograde flow of blood from the left ventricle into the atrium. Corresponding to the degree of valve damage, a portion of the left ventricular pressure is transmitted to the left atrium and thence back into the pulmonary bed. Since a portion of the cardiac stroke volume is lost through the mitral valve, the left ventricle enlarges to increase stroke volume and maintain an adequate peripheral circulation. The left atrium enlarges due to the increased pressure transmitted from the left ventricle. As the mitral valve becomes more insufficient, there is more enlargement of the left ventricle and atrium with additional corresponding changes in the lung fields. When sufficient retardation of blood flow in the pulmonary bed has occurred, enlargement of the right ventricle may develop. Roentgenographically, then, one could surmise that the left atrium would be much larger in mitral insufficiency than in mitral stenosis and that there is an enlargement of the left ventricle in mitral insufficiency which is generally not seen in pure mitral stenosis.

Long-standing mitral valve disease may produce a rather striking change in the cardiac silhouette as noted on the roentgenogram. In some patients with combined mitral insufficiency and mitral stenosis (Figs. 11-8, 11-9), the size of the cardiac silhouette may be great enough to occupy a large portion of the entire thorax. Conversely, changes may be only slight so that the mitral disease can only be surmised by the detection of calcium deposits within the mitral valve during fluoroscopy without a concomitant or previous history of rheumatic fever obtainable from the patient. The presence of calcification within the mitral valve is, therefore, secondary evidence of the presence of rheumatic heart disease, with or without a previous history of rheumatic fever.

Aortic valvular disease may present with no roentgen findings; and when findings are present, they are usually located in the aortic arch and left ventricle. Changes in the left ventricle are late findings, since the changes are primarily those of hypertrophy rather than dilatation. Changes in the aortic arch are related to pressure changes and flow patterns of the blood. In aortic stenosis (Fig. 11-10) there is a relative narrowing of the jet of blood as it leaves the aortic valve, and this jet of blood strikes against the anterolateral portion of the aortic arch, causing dilatation of the entire area which may extend up to the takeoff of the innominate vessel. In contrast, in aortic insufficiency there is a to-and-fro movement of the blood throughout the entire aortic arch due to a higher than normal cardiac output and to retrograde flow back across the insufficient valve. The roentgenographic changes therefore are limited to the entire arch rather than to the postvalvular area. The hallmark, therefore, of aortic stenosis is poststenotic dilatation of the aortic arch in the first portion of the arch. Dilatation of the entire arch is consistent with aortic insufficiency. As a person ages there is a normal uncoiling of the aortic arch, and it may be difficult in older patients to distinguish between the changes seen in aortic insufficiency and the normal uncoiling of the aortic arch and descending aorta. As in mitral valve disease, fluoroscopy may be of some benefit in diagnosing calcification

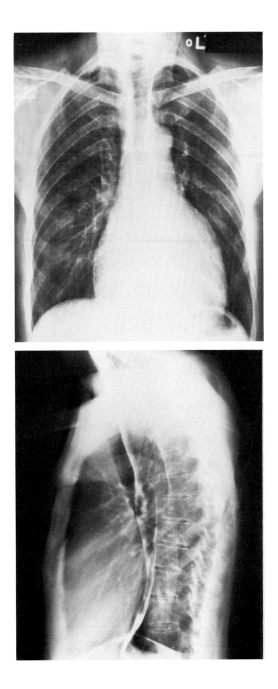

Fig. 11-8.
Combined mitral stenosis and insufficiency, moderately severe at cardiac catheterization.

within the valve or annulus. It may be extremely difficult to distinguish between calcific aortitis and a calcified aortic valve secondary to rheumatic heart disease.

Involvement of the tricuspid and pulmonary valves is infrequent in rheumatic heart disease, although it has been reported. Involvement of these valves is more likely to be of congenital origin than from an infectious process. Functional pulmonary and tricuspid insufficiency are not infrequent in the presence of severe mitral stenosis.

Bacterial endocarditis can occur, particularly in patients having borderline clinical mitral stenosis. The presence of vegetations on the valve may be sources for emboli into the systemic circulation with resultant infarction of tissue, leuko-cytosis, and fever. Hemoptysis is another clinical symptom that is seen in severe mitral stenosis. Table 11-1 summarizes the roentgenographic changes seen in rheumatic heart disease.

Table 11-1

Roentgenographic Changes in Rheumatic Heart Disease

	Atrium			Ventricle		
	L	R		L		R
M I	+ → 4+	0 → +		0 → 4+		0 → +
M S	+ → 2+	0 → +				0 → 2+
A I	0 → +	0		0 → 2+		0 (dilated aortic arch)
A S	0	0		0 → +		0 (poststenotic dilatation)
M I / M S	+ → 4+	0 → +		+ → 2+		0 → 2+
A I / A S	0	0		+ → 3+		0

MI = mitral insufficiency; MS = mitral stenosis; AI = aortic insufficiency; AS = aortic stenosis.

Congestive Heart Failure. As mentioned previously, the function of the heart is to supply a sufficient amount of blood to meet the metabolic requirements of tissue. If the heart cannot meet these requirements, heart failure is then said to exist. It is beyond the scope of this presentation to go into detail concerning the causes of cardiac failure, but these may be summarized as listed below:

1. Venous intake is greater than arterial output, as occurs, for example, in arteriovenous shunt or increased blood volume
2. Tissue demands increase above the cardiac output reserve, as occurs, for example, in thyrotoxicosis or sepsis
3. Decreased cardiac filling, as occurs, for example, secondary to constrictive pericarditis or valvular disease
4. Cardiac standstill

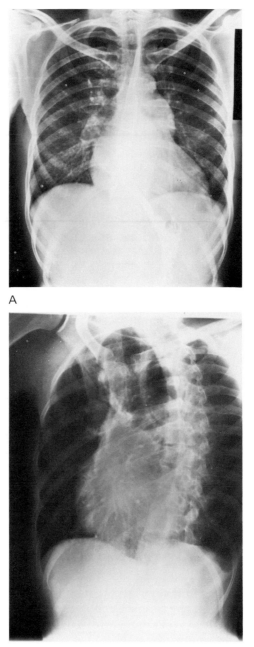

A

B

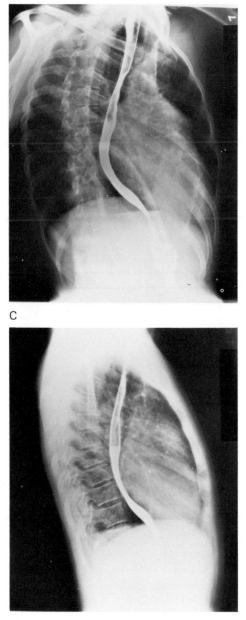

C

D

Fig. 11-9.

(A—D) Mild mitral stenosis, severe mitral insufficiency, and mild aortic insufficiency. Notice the double density behind the right heart on the PA film (A), indicating left atrial enlargement. Sometimes left atrial enlargement may also elevate the left main-stem bronchus, which is another indication of enlargement of the left atrium. The enlargement of the left atrial appendage obliterates the left pulmonary artery segment. On the LAO film (B) the appendage encroaches upon the pulmonary window.

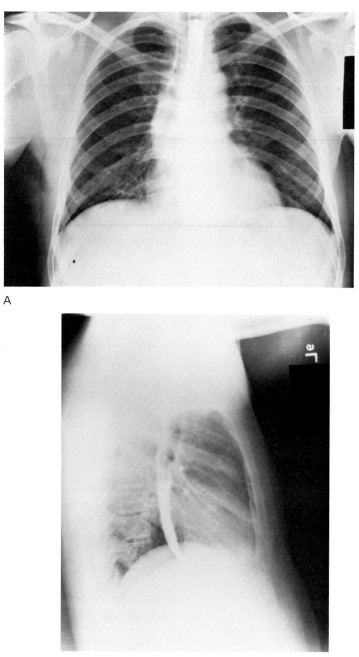

A

B

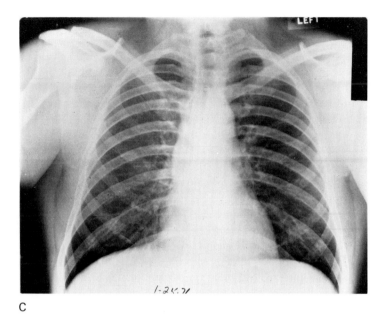

C

Fig. 11-10.

(A, B) Pure aortic stenosis. Notice the prominent poststenotic dilatation of the ascending aorta. The heart is enlarged, which is a late manifestation of aortic stenosis. (C) Two years after aortic valve replacement.

Left heart failure occurs when the left ventricle fails to pump a volume of blood equal to the venous return to the right ventricle. The left side of the heart may compensate for this deficiency by increasing cardiac rate, increasing stroke volume, or both. If these mechanisms do not compensate for the disparity between input and output, relative stasis of blood occurs with a resultant increase in pulmonary venous pressure and, passively, an increase in pulmonary artery pressure. Engorgement of the pulmonary veins ensues and the increased pressure allows tissue fluid to leak from capillaries into the interstitial tissues. As fluid in the interstitial spaces progresses, there is a point at which fluid actually enters the alveolar and bronchial components of the lung, producing audible rales and subsequently pleural effusion.

In right heart failure, blood accumulates on the venous side of the circulation producing engorgement of the vena cavae, liver enlargement, and pitting edema of the lower extremities.

Clinical manifestations of congestive heart failure vary according to the severity and acuteness of the failure. In left heart failure, manifestations are primarily respiratory in nature, with the patient complaining of dyspnea. In right heart failure the patient's chief complaint is that of ankle swelling which disappears overnight. He may also complain of anorexia or indigestion, which result from concomitant hepatic enlargement.

Roentgenographically (Fig. 11-11), one of the most common changes seen on the film is an increase in heart size. It should be noted at this time that the heart size may increase from its normal standard and still appear within normal limits roentgenographically, so one must compare cardiac size to that which has been known previously. For example, if the cardiothoracic ratio was 38 percent on a previous examination and on the current examination measures 48 percent, there has indeed been a rather marked increase in cardiac size, although the cardiac enlargement is still within normal limits. As a general rule the cardiac enlargement is much more marked than the example above and may be quite obvious on the roentgenogram. As the pressure in the left atrium increases, the pressure is transmitted back through the pulmonary veins with resultant engorgement of the veins and prominence of the hilar vessels, so the normal convexed appearance of the hilar vessels becomes concave. In addition, the transverse pulmonary vein that empties directly into the center of the hilar area may become engorged, helping to create the concave appearance of the hilum. As failure increases, there is a constriction of the vessels of the lower lung field with

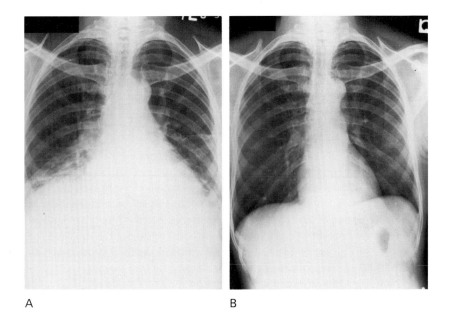

A   B

Fig. 11-11.

(A) Congestive heart failure with pulmonary edema and bilateral pleural effusion. Notice the prominent pulmonary vessels in the hila and upper lung fields. (B) Same patient three weeks later.

a resultant dilatation of the vessels in the upper lung field, so that one then sees what is called a pulmonary vascular shift; this may be one of the first signs that one can detect in congestive heart failure. As the failure increases there is escape of fluid into the interstitial spaces, presenting on the roentgenogram as a butterfly-shaped collection of fluid around the hilar areas. With further increase in failure, frank fluffy infiltrates will appear throughout the lung fields. As these increase, pleural effusion may be produced, generally first on the right and then on the left. If right heart failure is also present there is almost inevitably an increase in tissue fluid in the soft tissues, particularly the skin, as noted by pitting edema in the pretibial areas. This may be seen on the roentgenogram as loss of the thoracic fat stripes, as the fluid is retained within the fat spaces between the muscle layers of the chest.

As congestive heart failure recedes there is resorption of the pleural effusion and clearing of the lung fields. This is associated with a decrease in the cardiac size and eventually a shift of the blood vessels back to a normal size.

Arteriosclerotic Heart Disease. Arteriosclerotic heart disease occurs secondary to the deposition of atheromatous plaques within the coronary arteries to such a degree that myocardial damage or ischemia results (Fig. 11-12). As plaque deposition increases, myocardial infarction may occur with subsequent necrosis of muscle and replacement with fibrous tissue. The area of the infarction may heal with little subsequent physical disability; or a ventricular aneurysm may develop, with all shades of variation in between. Dystrophic calcification may also occur in the region of the infarction.

Roentgenographically, the radiologist may see no change referable to arteriosclerotic heart disease. As the patient ages, mild increase in heart size may occur which may be detected roentgenographically. At fluoroscopy, calcific deposits may be seen in the coronary arteries. Although not consistently present, tortuosity of the aorta and great vessels with calcific deposits in the aortic arch may be noted. As the heart exceeds its cardiac reserve, frank manifestations of cardiac failure may be seen roentgenographically. These changes are essentially the same as have been described above under Congestive Heart Failure.

Hypertensive Heart Disease. Hypertensive vascular disease is perhaps the most common cause of congestive heart failure seen in the adult at about the age of 55 to 60 years. Hypertensive heart disease occurs when the cardiac reserve is expended against an increased peripheral resistance. This type of heart disease may be associated with myocardial ischemia as clinically signified by the presence of angina and myocardial infarction, or it may occur with no clinically significant cardiac changes.

Since the clinical course of hypertensive cardiovascular disease is such that it may be years before cardiac changes become manifest, roentgenographic changes are usually limited to the appearance of cardiac enlargement in the older or

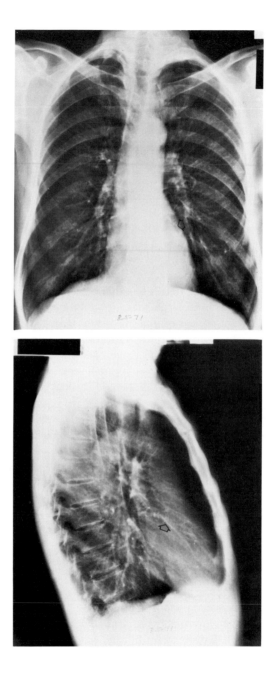

Fig. 11-12.
 Arteriosclerotic heart disease and coronary artery calcification. This patient had severe heart disease and died a few days after these films were made. The cardiac size is normal.

geriatric patient. As the cardiac condition worsens, the picture of congestive heart failure will appear and present roentgenographically as noted previously (Fig. 11-13).

PERICARDIAL EFFUSION

The major causes of pericardial effusion include tuberculosis and viral infections. On occasion one may see effusion secondary to invasion of the pericardium by malignant tumors, chronic renal failure, or myocardial infarction. The pericardial effusion may be of a mild degree and have no essential clinical significance, or the fluid may be accumulated to such an extent that the heart is constricted in its motion with resultant cardiac tamponade. Although there are several good ways to demonstrate pericardial effusion, perhaps one of the most accurate is through the use of ultrasonography.

Roentgenographically, the presence of pericardial effusion may be suspected by the rather rapid increase in heart size without concomitant signs of cardiac failure (Fig. 11-14). Sometimes one may see a posteriorly displaced substernal subepicardial fat line, which is indicative of pericardial effusion; and on occasion the right cardiophrenic angle may become more acute than is normally seen, which also suggests the presence of effusion. However, it is generally conceded that the diagnosis of pericardial effusion is suspected clinically and demonstrated roentgenographically by the use of angiography. Demonstration of thickness of the right ventricle is accomplished by injecting contrast material into the right atrium and measuring the thickness of the wall. In addition, one may inject carbon dioxide into the right atrium in the left lateral decubitus view to demonstrate increased thickness of the extraluminal band. Ultrasonography is accomplished by bouncing sound waves off the interspaces between the fluid of the epicardium and the pericardium and measuring the distance. In the normal state there should be no appreciable space between the epicardium and pericardium; and in the presence of fluid this space will widen. Thus, since the fluid will conduct sound, this area can be measured and a fairly accurate estimation made of the amount of fluid within the pericardial sac.

AORTIC ARCH

Signs and symptoms referable to infirmities involving the aortic arch may be subclinical, subtle, or protean. Most congenital anomalies of the arch are first diagnosed in the pediatric age group and are observed in adult patients at follow-up examinations. The common congenital anomalies include aortic atresia, coarctation, stenosis, patent ductus arteriosus, transposition of the great vessels, and tetralogy of Fallot. Anomalies of the innominate and subclavian vessels may

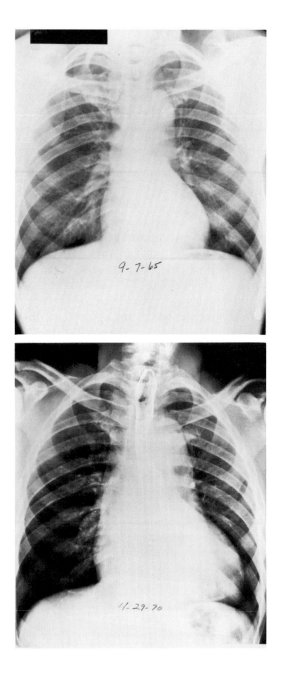

Fig. 11-13.

Hypertensive cardiovascular disease. This patient ultimately developed a dissecting aneurysm of the aorta some five years later. Notice the tortuous aorta noted in 1965 and the marked changes in 1970.

290

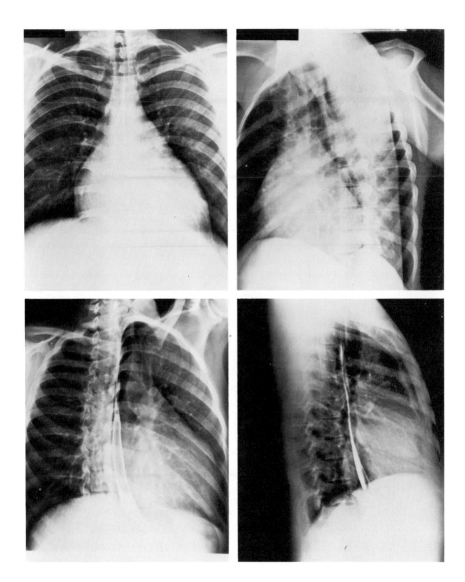

Fig. 11-14.

Pericardial effusion. Notice the globe-shaped heart silhouette and relatively avascular lung fields. Although the cardiac silhouette is enlarged, there is no appreciable deviation of the esophagus.

create so-called vascular rings and produce swallowing and respiratory distress by compression of the esophagus or trachea. However, the most common diseases affecting the aorta in the adult patient are aortic aneurysm and atherosclerotic changes. Developmental anomalies such as pseudocoarctation (Fig. 11-15) and right-sided aortic arch (Fig. 11-16) do occur and must be recognized.

Arteriosclerosis occurs secondary to deposition of circulatory lipids in the intima of the aortic wall. Other contributory factors include the normal aging process, hypertension, and possible degeneration of the vasa vasorum — the small nutrient vessels supplying the aortic wall. Arteriosclerosis per se is symptomless, and only until a small artery supplying an organ is occluded or a vessel wall is ruptured will signs and symptoms present. It is a rather common finding, being seen in many asymptomatic patients (Fig. 11-17).

Aortic aneurysms are of three types: fusiform, dissecting, and saccular. Dissecting aneurysms (Figs. 11-18, 11-19) are usually associated with hypertension and begin in the aortic arch, extending a variable distance along the aorta. Excruciating chest pain may accompany dissecting aneurysms, and sudden hemiplegia may result from occlusion of carotid vessels. Differentiation from myocardial infarction must be considered, and one valuable point to recognize is that patients with dissecting aneurysms may have high blood pressures as compared to relatively low pressures in patients with myocardial infarction. Serial roentgenography may demonstrate the dissection. Other thoracic or mediastinal masses should also be considered.

Saccular and fusiform aneurysms occur more commonly in the distal abdominal aorta, celiac artery, and popliteal artery. As with dissecting aneurysms, pain may be the presenting symptom; but most of these aneurysms are palpable either by the patient or the physician when examining the area for other reasons.

There are obviously other major diseases involving the heart and great vessels such as mycotic aneurysms of the aorta, congenital malformations such as coarctation, and the whole realm of pediatric congenital heart diseases. In actual practice, congenital heart disease is relatively rare; and a study of these lesions should be undertaken by those who have a particular interest in pediatric cardiology.

If the student can appreciate from the foregoing discussion how the normal cardiac silhouette should appear and some of the possibilities when the cardiac silhouette is enlarged, a large portion of the battle for understanding may be won. It is generally not the prerogative of the student to make the diagnosis, but it should be within the prerogatives of allied health personnel to suggest to the physician that an abnormality may exist.

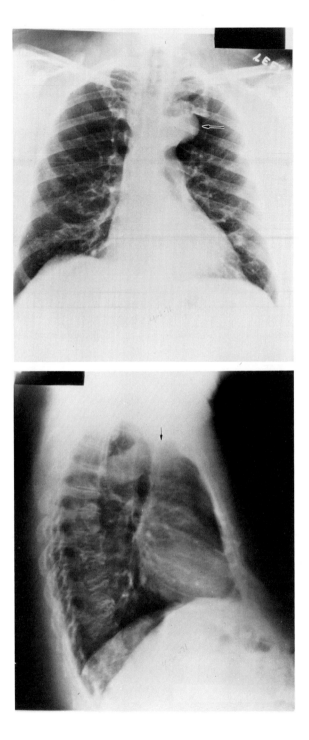

Fig. 11-15.

Pseudocoarctation of the aorta. This was a preemployment chest film of an asymptomatic patient. Notice the prominent aortic knob on the PA film and prominent buckling on the lateral film.

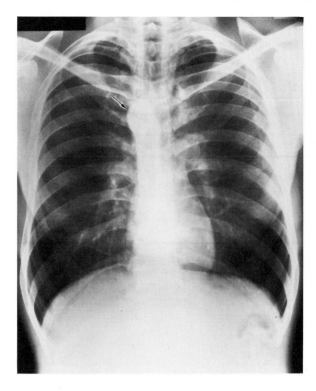

Fig. 11-16.
Right-sided aortic arch in an asymptomatic patient.

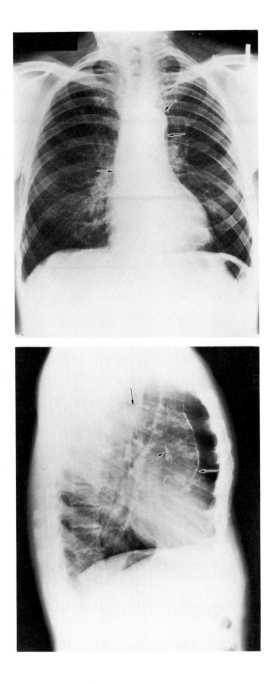

Fig. 11-17.
    Heavy arteriosclerotic calcification of the aorta. The calcification is seen better on the lateral than on the PA film.

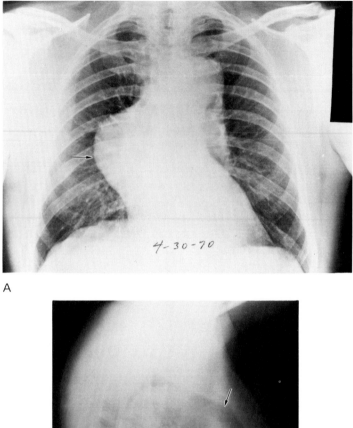

A

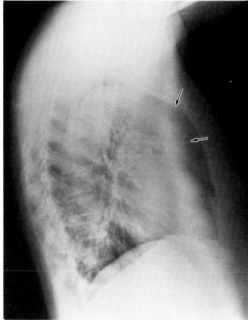

B

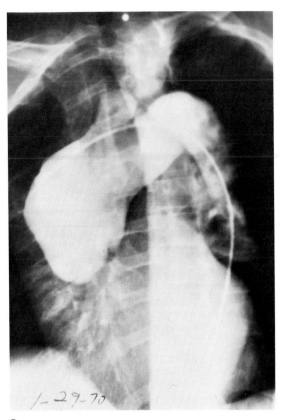

C

Fig. 11-18.
(A, B) Dissecting aortic aneurysm beginning at the level of the aortic valve. (C) An angiogram demonstrates the size of the aneurysm as compared to the size of the normal descending aorta.

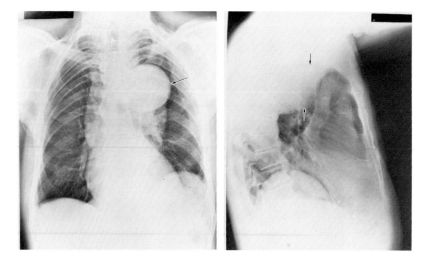

Fig. 11-19.
    Fusiform aortic aneurysms beginning in the aortic arch and extending to the level of the renal arteries. This aneurysm did not change in appearance over a six-year period.

READING LIST

General

Edwards, J. E., Cary, L. S., Neufield, H. N., and Lester, R. G. *Congenital Heart Disease.*
        Philadelphia: Saunders, 1965.
Friedberg, C. K. *Diseases of the Heart,* 3d ed., vol. 1. Philadelphia: Saunders, 1966.
Taussig, H. B. *Congenital Malformations of the Heart.* New York: Commonwealth Fund,
        1947.

Specific

Elliott, L. P. (Ed.). Radiology of the Heart. *Radiol. Clin. North Am.* vol. 6, no. 3, 1968.
Hipona, F. A. (Ed.). Cardiac Radiology: Surgical Aspects. *Radiol. Clin. North Am.* vol. 9,
        no. 2, 1971.
Hipona, F. A. (Ed.). Cardiac Radiology: Medical Aspects. *Radiol. Clin. North Am.* vol. 9,
        no. 3, 1971.

Nuclear Medicine

12

DURING THE PAST TWO DECADES we have witnessed a rapid growth in the field of nuclear medicine. From a fragmented service run by pathologists, internists, and radiologists a few years ago, nuclear medicine has become a full-fledged specialty with its own Board certification. This phenomenal growth is due to an increased accessibility to radiopharmaceuticals, improved instrumentation, simple administration of tests, low morbidity, and the clinician's awareness of the value of radionuclide tests.

Before considering the clinical applications of nuclear medicine, some of the terms commonly used in the specialty should be defined.

Radionuclide (Radioisotope). Generally the radioactive counterpart of a normally occurring element. The radioactive element has an unstable nucleus and, in attempting to become stable, emits small bits of energized particles called *alpha* or *beta rays* or energy such as gamma or roentgen rays. Most radionuclide scans utilize gamma emission. The different isotopes of a given element are conventionally identified by citation of their characteristic mass number. Normal iodine, for example, is mass number 127 and is written iodine 127 or ^{127}I; the most common radioactive isotope of iodine has a mass of 131 and is abbreviated as ^{131}I.

Radiopharmaceutical. Contains a radionuclide which is used for localization or measurement or both. May be used for diagnostic procedures or therapy. In diagnostic studies produces no pharmaceutical effect.

Physical Half-life. The time required for a radioactive element to disintegrate to 50 percent of the original number of atoms.

Effective Half-life. The time required for 50 percent of the radiopharmaceutical to be eliminated from the body by body excretion and physical decay.

Biological Half-life. The time required for 50 percent of the radiopharmaceutical to be excreted or secreted from the body, usually in feces or urine.

299

Curie. 3.7 × 10¹⁰ nuclear disintegrations per second.

Millicurie. 1/1,000 of a curie, abbreviated mCi.

Microcurie. One-millionth of a curie, abbreviated μCi.

Generator (Cow). Contains a long-lived isotope (parent) which decays to produce a clinically useful, short half-life radioisotope (daughter).

Scan. Produces a two-dimensional picture of an organ and tends to provide a faithful reproduction of radioactivity distributed within an organ:

1. *Rectilinear scan.* Systematic recording of radioactive information by a detector containing a 3 or 5 inch sodium iodide crystal which longitudinally indexes across an organ (Fig. 12-1).
2. *Scintillation camera.* Systematic recording of radioactivity by a stationary detector (usually an 11- or 12-inch sodium iodide crystal) (Fig. 12-2).

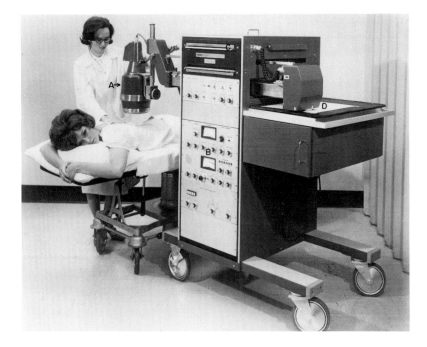

Fig. 12-1.

Picker Nuclear Magnascanner 500, a rectilinear scanner. In simplified terms, radiation from the patient is detected and converted to electronic signals at point A. At point B the electronic signals are amplified and indexed and displayed on film (C) and paper (D). The film is developed through a standard radiographic processing machine to produce images such as are noted in this chapter. The rectilinear scanner is versatile and useful in most nuclear medicine laboratories. (Photo courtesy Picker Nuclear, Cleveland, Ohio.)

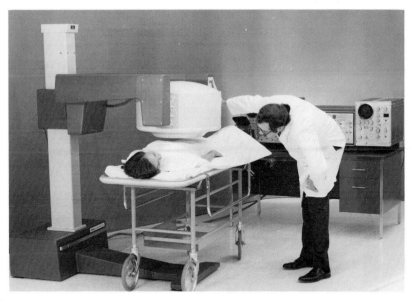

Fig. 12-2.
Picker Nuclear Dynacamera, a scintillation camera. This mechanism is essentially the same as the rectilinear scanner except the detector is much larger and does not move back and forth across the patient. Images are projected on an oscilloscope and are then photographed to produce dynamic or static isotopic studies. (Photo courtesy Picker Nuclear, Cleveland, Ohio.)

Radiopharmaceutical is commonly used interchangeably with the terms *tracer,* *radioisotope,* and *radionuclide.* A tracer ideally should consist of an isotope with a long enough physical and biological half-life that a procedure can be performed and yet produce an insignificant or acceptable amount of radiation damage to the patient. One prefers not to use beta- or alpha-emitting isotopes, as these particles produce tissue damage without significantly contributing to a diagnosis. However, one of the most commonly used isotopes, ^{131}I, produces beta emission; and a pure beta emitter (radioactive phosphorus, ^{32}P) is used in therapy of polycythemia.

Tracers can be localized within an organ according to the following basic mechanisms:

1. *Active transport.* The isotope is absorbed and utilized exactly as its non-radioactive companion, e.g., the use of ^{131}I in thyroid uptake and scanning.
2. *Exchange diffusion.* The isotope is substituted for another element of similar chemical property, e.g., strontium 85 is utilized in active bone formation in place of calcium and can be detected by scanning.

3. *Phagocytosis.* Here the isotope is ingested by the reticuloendothelial system, particularly within the spleen and liver, e.g., liver scanning with technetium-labeled sulfide colloid.
4. *Cell sequestration.* Accumulation within an organ of damaged cells prelabeled with a radioisotope, e.g., spleen scanning with heat-damaged ^{51}Cr-labeled red blood cells.
5. *Capillary block.* Formation of microemboli in small capillaries, e.g., lung scanning with macroaggregated albumin I 131.
6. *Compartmental localization.* Utilization of the knowledge that an organ contains a large amount of a body substance which lends itself to being tagged with a tracer, e.g., heart blood pool scanning or placental scanning with technetium-labeled albumin.

Obviously some organs can be examined by using a combination of the mechanisms described above. For example, the heart blood pool can be examined by the use of technetium-labeled albumin and indirectly one can infer the cardiac size; or one can scan the myocardium itself with cesium 131 and get a direct visualization of the cardiac size. The same can be done with the liver by using sulfide colloid, Te 99m, which is ingested by reticuloendothelial cells, or one can use rose bengal I 131, which is actively concentrated by the liver parenchymal cells and excreted in bile.

In addition to scanning to visualize tracer uptake in organs, one can tag normal body constituents with tracers to determine their behavior within the body. Thus, red blood cells can be tagged with an isotope to determine their survival time within the body or protein can be labeled to evaluate loss or absorption from the gastrointestinal tract.

All these procedures have enhanced our diagnostic acumen and the understanding of physiological and pathological disease processes.

ORGAN SCANNING

Brain Scanning. The development of brain scanning has resulted in a significant advance in evaluation of intracranial disease. Rather than replacing any of the current nonradioisotopic neuroradiological examinations such as the pneumoencephalogram or carotid arteriogram, the brain scan is becoming an important addition to the physician's diagnostic procedures.

Initially the brain scan was used to locate and confirm neoplastic conditions within the cranial vault. The applications of brain scanning for lesions other than neoplasms soon became apparent, and scanning is now regarded as a frontline screening test for intracranial disease without appreciable patient hazard.

The most commonly used radiopharmaceutical in brain scanning is technetium 99m pertechnetate. Radioiodinated human serum albumin Hg 197 and chlormerodrin Hg 203 have been used previously, but [203]Hg has now been declared out of bounds for brain scanning by the Atomic Energy Commission. The advantage of using mercury for brain scanning is that the compound has a long shelf life as compared to the half-life of six hours for technetium. In some institutions, indium 113m, another generator-produced radionuclide, is also used for brain scanning.

No preparation is necessary for adult patients; but in children, Lugol's solution or saturated potassium iodide is usually given 24 hours prior to the scan to reduce radiation to the thyroid gland. In some departments potassium perchlorate may be given orally about an hour prior to the scan to reduce uptake in the thyroid gland, choroid plexus, salivary glands, and stomach, all of which are known to concentrate the pertechnetate ion.

At least four views of the brain are taken following the intravenous administration of the radiopharmaceutical. Normal scans (Fig. 12-3) reveal high concentrations of the radiopharmaceutical in the vascular spaces of the cranium. There is heavy uptake in the region of the salivary glands, as is seen on almost all scans. In the occipital area there is an increased uptake in the region where the superior sagittal sinus and transverse sinuses form an area called the *torcula herophili.*

Cerebral necrosis such as that occurring in cerebral malacia, abscesses, or intracranial hematoma will have a positive scan. In patients with cerebral vascular accident the brain scan is usually positive after seven to ten days, returning to normal after approximately four weeks. Serial scans show improvement which usually supersedes or at least parallels clinical improvement. Subdural hematomas show increased uptake in the reactive membrane. Arteriovenous malformations usually have positive scans if the patient has an associated intracranial or intracerebral bleeding.

The privilege of using the brain scan as a screening test must carry with it the obligation on the part of the interpreter or physician who requests the test to understand the limitations and pitfalls of the procedure. This is graphically illustrated by the fact that the brain scan is notoriously negative for small, slow-growing intracranial neoplasms which carry with them the potential for resection and cure. To allow the misinterpretation of a "normal" brain scan as absolutely ruling out such a neoplasm would be unfortunate. Poorly differentiated astrocytomas or oligodendrogliomas and meningiomas are well seen on the scan. Well-differentiated or diffuse infiltrative tumors are less well seen and may have negative scans. Metastases greater than 1 cm in diameter are usually outlined.

Not infrequently the scan is positive when more hazardous procedures such as cerebral angiography and air studies are negative or normal. Conversely, the opposite may also be true, as the brain scan complements rather than replaces these procedures. For equivocal scans it is often necessary to repeat the procedure using a second radiopharmaceutical with different clearance rates and concentration or to delay the scan for two to three hours after the administration of technetium 99m.

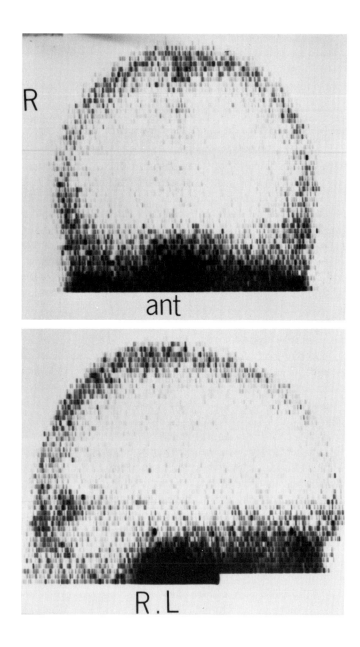

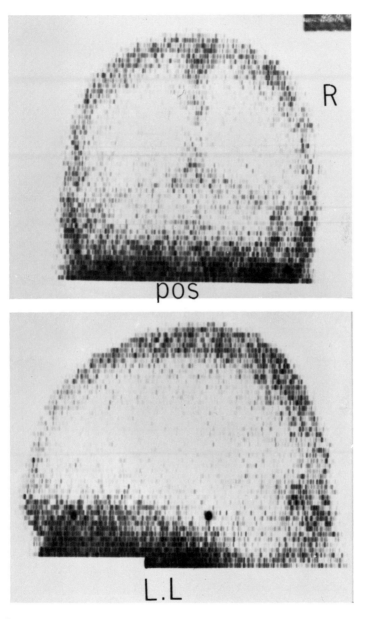

Fig. 12-3.
Normal four-view brain scan. Notice how uniform the tracer activity is over the soft tissues of the cranium. There is no activity in the brain substance itself.

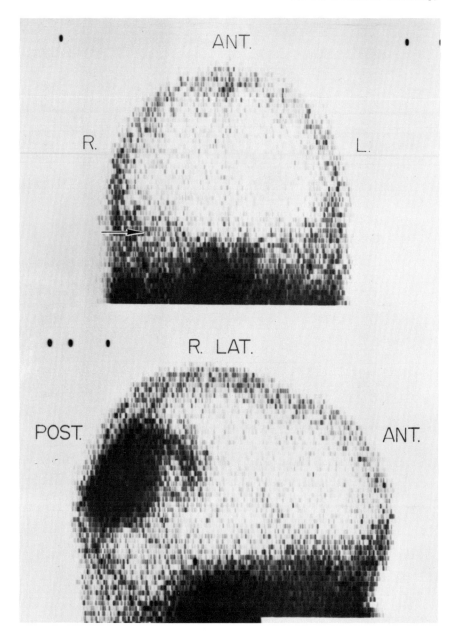

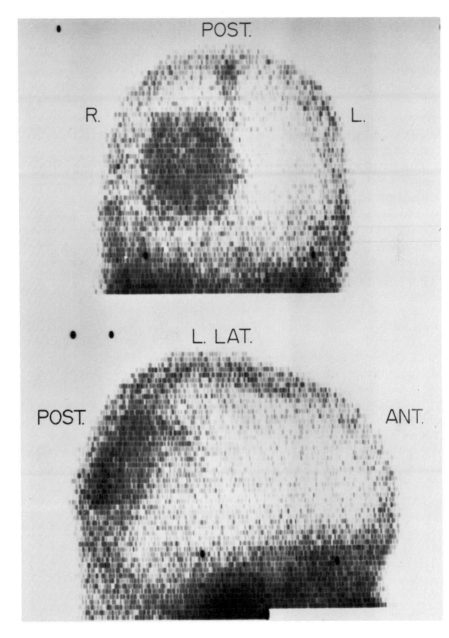

Fig. 12-4.

   In this four-view brain scan there is a gross uptake in a lesion located in the right posterior parietal area. On the anterior view there is only a slight increase in activity noted at arrow. As in diagnostic roentgenography, multiple views are necessary to prevent overlooking a lesion.

An abnormal concentration of the tracer in pathological areas is due to a change in the blood—brain permeability, although in some cases it is probably related primarily to an increased vascularity of the lesion, such as occurs in arteriovenous malformations. When there is no change in the vascularity or the blood—brain permeability, the brain scan is usually normal, since the radiocompound generally is confined to the cerebral intravascular spaces. One may then state that in the abnormal brain scan or in any other scan, an abnormal amount of the radiocompound is concentrated within the diseased area; and in normal areas the concentration is normal.

Interpretation of brain scans is primarily that of any other area in radiology, namely by the establishment of symmetry. By comparing one view to another and one part of the particular scan to another, one can pick up minor alterations which may turn a negative study into a positive one, or vice versa. Figure 12-3 is a normal brain scan, and Figure 12-4 presents a grossly positive scan. Gradations between the two exist in actual practice.

In summary, one may say that the brain scan is an accurate screening examination which complements other roentgenographic procedures and in turn presents essentially no hazard to the patient.

Lung Scanning. As the student may remember from pulmonary physiology, the lung consists of many ordered bronchi and air sacs. Adjacent to these tubes and sacs are pulmonary arteries ranging in size from 15 mm to about 6μ. These arterioles are distributed uniformly throughout the lungs but are perfused differently according to cardiac dynamics and position of the patient.

By injecting foreign particulate matter which is filtered within the pulmonary capillary bed, one can examine lung perfusion with little or no patient morbidity. The particulate matter acts as short-lived microemboli which are ultimately phagocytized by the reticuloendothelial cells. However, only a minute fraction of the capillaries is embolized, and this procedure produces no detectable alteration in pulmonary function.

In the presence of pulmonary pathology such as thromboembolization, emphysema, carcinoma, pneumonia, and so on, there may be an area of decreased perfusion of the affected area, producing an area of decreased radioactivity on the perfusion scan. Scans must be interpreted in the presence of a chest roentgenogram taken during the same time span and in the same position as the scan was made. An abnormal scan in the presence of a normal chest roentgenogram is significant. Abnormal areas of a scan compatible to areas of abnormality on a chest roentgenogram are not a conclusive diagnosis of emboli but, at the same time, cannot exclude emboli.

In most nuclear medicine departments, four views of the chest are obtained during a lung scan. These include an AP, PA, and both lateral projections. The scan is then compared to chest roentgenograms, with abnormal areas on the scan compared to the same areas on the chest films.

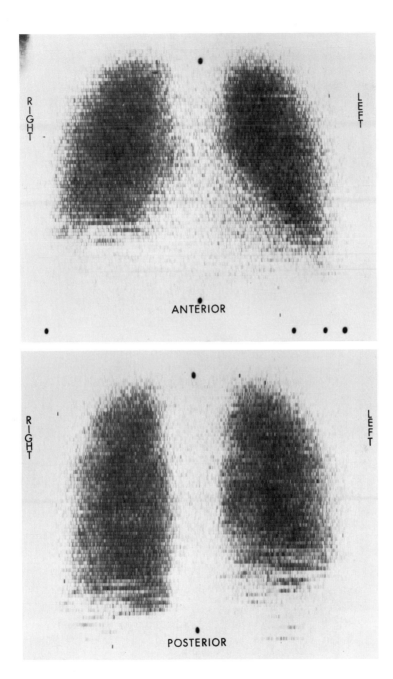

RIGHT

LEFT

ANTERIOR

RIGHT

LEFT

POSTERIOR

Fig. 12-5.

Normal lung scan. Activity in the lower lung fields is decreased because of respiratory motion. Notice that more lung volume is detected on the posterior scan than on the anterior scan.

Anterior lung

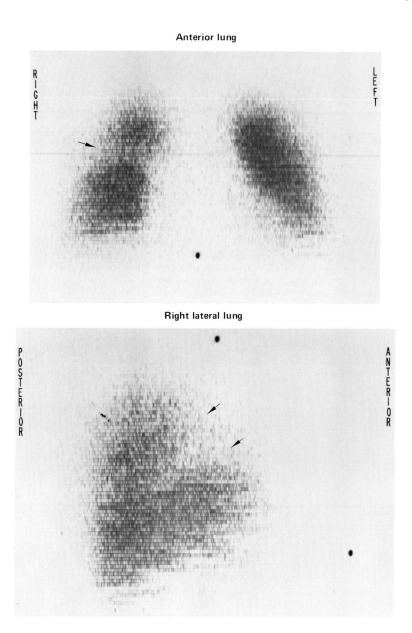

Right lateral lung

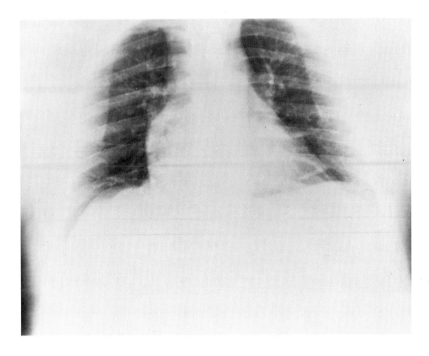

Fig. 12-6.
   Lung scans of a pulmonary embolus in the anterior segment of the right upper lobe. There
is no pathology in the same area noted on the chest film.

   Note should be made concerning the criteria for the particulate matter used
for the lung scan. In order to have a useful scan the particles must be of uniform
size and radioactivity. Complete intravascular mixing must occur before perfusion of the lung in order to have complete uniformity throughout the bases
and apices of the lungs. The absolute essential to using tagged particles for lung
scanning is that they must be extracted or filtered within the pulmonary capillary
bed on the first passage through the lung parenchyma. A short-circuiting of the
particles may lead to embolization to the brain or other organs of the body;
therefore, any patient with cardiac shunt should not have a lung scan.
   Lung scanning can be complemented by pulmonary angiography. This is
particularly useful when the lung scan is positive, for example, in pulmonary
emphysema one may have to exclude the possibility of pulmonary emboli.
Hence the pulmonary angiogram may be helpful in differentiating areas of
abnormal scans in the presence of an abnormal chest roentgenogram. Figure
12-5 is a normal lung scan as compared to the pulmonary embolus shown in
Figure 12-6.

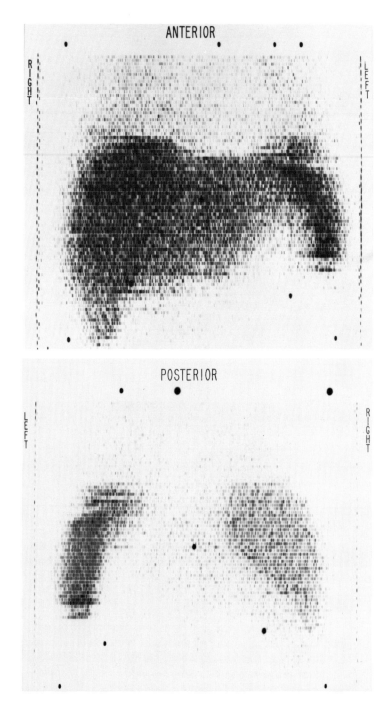

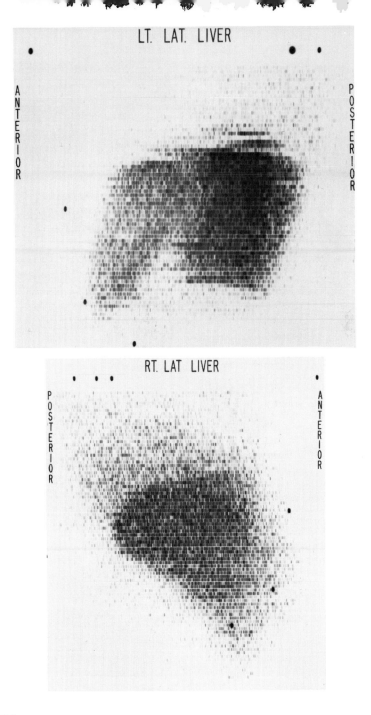

Fig. 12-7.

Normal four-view liver scan. On the anterior scan there is about uniform activity of the tracer in the spleen and liver. Since the spleen is more posterior, there is more activity over the spleen than over the liver on the posterior scan, which is again confirmed on the left lateral views. The spleen is masked by liver activity on the right lateral view.

313

Liver Scanning. It was mentioned in the introduction that one of the mechanisms of localizing radionuclides is phagocytosis. Liver scanning uses this principle in determining the size, shape, and location of the liver. The patient is given an intravenous injection of technetium-labeled sulfide colloid which is rapidly phagocytized by the Kupffer cells of the liver. Since the Kupffer cells are distributed uniformly throughout the liver, one can obtain a uniform uptake of the tracer throughout the liver. Any space-occupying lesion greater than about 2 cm in diameter will appear as a "hole," or area of decreased activity in the silhouette of the liver. Only with an adequate medical history can one ascertain what the area of decreased uptake may be. For example, if single or multiple areas of decreased activity are present on the liver scan and the patient has carcinoma, one might presume that the areas of decreased activity represent metastases. However, if the patient has had septicemia followed by a fever of unknown origin, one might conclude that the areas of decreased activity represent multiple abscesses.

By changing isotopes and using rose bengal I 131, the same information as noted above can be obtained. However, by obtaining delayed scans, the biliary tree can be differentiated from the liver parenchyma, thus adding another important test for diagnosis of disease.

When colloids are used for liver scanning, an auxiliary finding is that of depiction of the size, shape, and position of the spleen. Also, liver scans may be utilized in conjunction with lung scanning to show the presence of subdiaphragmatic abscesses or space-occupying lesions located between the lung and liver. Figures 12-7 through 12-10 represent typical changes seen on liver scans.

Liver scanning may show the size, shape, and position of the liver and spleen. As in all scanning, the presence of a positive scan is significant and "normal" scans may be misleading.

Other Organs. A few comments should be made concerning imaging of other organs. Scanning of the liver, lung, spleen, and brain are by far the most common images recorded; but other scans also have importance. Cisternography scanning is performed by instilling a labeled human serum albumin intrathecally. The albumin normally diffuses to the basal cisterns and subarachnoid space and is eventually absorbed within 48 hours. This examination is useful in evaluating cerebrospinal leaks and low-pressure hydrocephalus and is commonly used by neurosurgeons in evaluating patients for possible shunt operations.

Scanning of the skeletal system with ^{99m}Tc polyphosphate, ^{18}F, and ^{85}Sr is used to demonstrate increased bone activity. Bone scans are useful in determining areas of metastatic tumor, since scans usually detect positive changes earlier than do roentgenograms. These scans are also useful in determining the extent of a lesion when bone roentgenograms are positive and in localizing radiotherapy portals. The scan is frequently positive months before lesions show on roentgenograms.

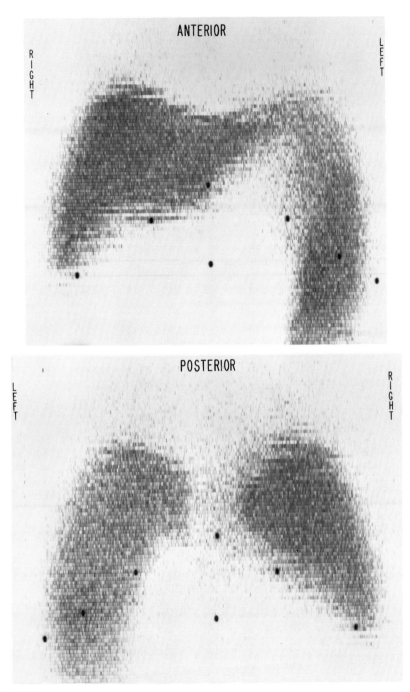

ANTERIOR

RIGHT

LEFT

POSTERIOR

LEFT

RIGHT

Fig. 12-8.
Liver scans in a 25-year-old patient with leukemia. There is a huge spleen which extended past the edge of the film and was palpable below the iliac crest.

315

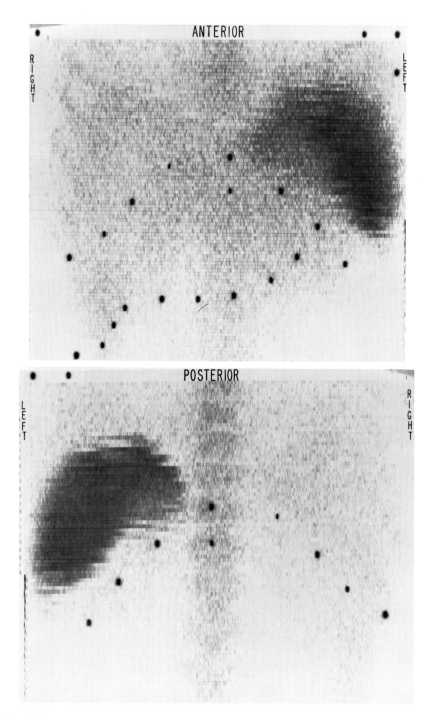

Fig. 12-9.

Huge liver with moderate increase in splenic size. This is the patchy distribution of far-advanced, diffuse hepatocellular disease.

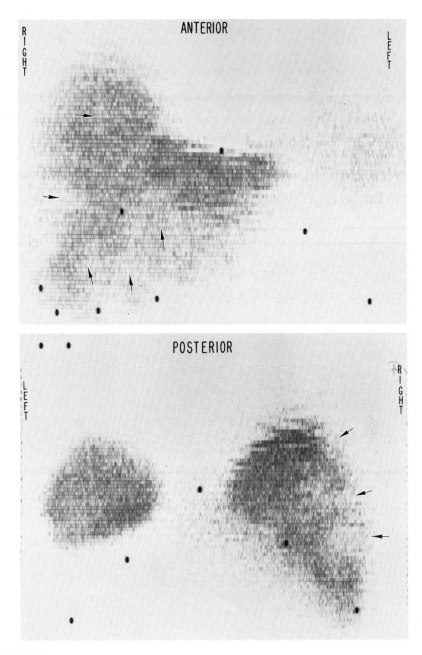

Fig. 12-10.

Metastatic carcinoma to the liver. Notice the large radiolucent filling defects in the liver, and compare to Figure 12-9.

Renal scans are performed using chlormerodrin Hg 197, which is bound to the renal tubules. Renal scans supplement roentgenographic studies and are commonly utilized when the kidneys are not visualized on an intravenous urogram or for localization of the kidney when other contrast studies are contraindicated.

Injection of large doses of radioactive substances will allow one to evaluate the cardiac or placental blood pool. In the chest, the greater amount of activity should correspond to the cardiac silhouette of a six-foot focus—film supine chest roentgenogram. If the area of activity is smaller than the heart size on the roentgenogram, pericardial effusion should be suspected. In placental localization, the same principle applies — the placenta is the most vascular structure within the bounds of the uterus. Care should be taken not to confuse bladder activity with a low-lying placenta or vice versa.

THE THYROID GLAND

Perhaps one of the most commonly requested examinations in nuclear medicine is evaluation of thyroid size, shape, and function. A variety of thyroid examinations are available to the clinician. Generally, these include thyroid uptake and thyroid scans, using ^{131}I as the principal tracer.

Thyroid Physiology. The function of the thyroid gland is to take inorganic iodide from plasma and convert it to organic iodine. It is combined with an amino acid, tyrosine, and finally converted to thyroid hormones, principally thyroxine (T_4) and triiodothyronine (T_3). The T_3 and T_4 are then combined with thyroglobulin and stored in the thyroid follicles. Under regulation, primarily by thyroid stimulatory hormone (TSH) from the anterior pituitary, hypothalamus, or plasma levels of thyroid, the hormones are broken down from the thyroglobulin by means of enzymatic proteolysis and are released into the bloodstream, mainly in the form of thyroxine (90 percent) and triiodothyronine (10 percent). The hormones are bound to plasma glycoproteins, termed *thyroxine-binding globulin* (TBG), *prealbumin* (TBPA), and *serum albumin.* A small amount of thyroxine is found free in the plasma.

The effects of thyroid hormones are manifold. Disorders of body function may occur as a consequence of either hypofunction or hyperfunction. Hypofunction may be related to changes in gland size and is most frequently due to goiter, adenoma, thyroiditis, or malignancies. Large glands produce symptoms secondary to compression in the neck and extension into the superior mediastinum. Abnormal hormone output affects cellular oxidation mechanisms, basal metabolic rate (BMR), pulse rate, and so on.

Factors Affecting Thyroid Function. Thyroid function is affected by so many different factors that it has become necessary to list specific drugs which a patient may be taking or may recently have taken in order to anticipate results from radioactive examinations effectively. Different drugs may block the iodine cycle at different points, but it is sufficient to state that the thyroid-trapping mechanism is enhanced by thyroid-stimulating hormone (TSH) and blocked by potassium thiocyanate drugs. Conversion into organic iodine (oxidation reaction) may be blocked by thiourea compounds of sulfonamides. Breakdown of the colloid thyroglobulin is enhanced by TSH and blocked by excessive levels of plasma iodine. Table 12-1 is a partial list of common medications which may affect thyroid uptake of iodine.

Table 12-1.

Factors Affecting Thyroid Radioiodine Uptake

Increase	*Decrease*	
1. Iodine-deficient diet	1. Iodine compounds	
2. Rebound from antithyroid drugs	X-ray contrast media studies (intravenous	
3. Cobalt hematinic	pyelogram, gallbladder, angiogram,	
4. Nephrosis	myelogram, bronchogram)	
5. Thyroid-stimulating hormone	Antiparasitic drugs	
	(Floraquin, Vioform)	
	Cough medicines	
	Vitamin preparations	
	Lugol's, ssKI (saturated solution potassium	
	iodide) (lung scan)	
	Suntan lotions	
	2. Thyroid medications	
	Tapazole, propylthiouracil	
	Thiocyanate, perchlorate (brain scan)	
	Thyroxine (Synthroid, etc.)	
	Cytomel	
No Effect	3. Miscellaneous drugs	
1. Oral contraceptives	Corticoids	Pentothal
2. Estrogens	ACTH	Orinase
3. Androgens	Salicylates	Sulfonamides
4. Phenobarbital	Phenylbutazone	PASA, INH
5. Reserpine	Thiazides	PABA
6. Mercurial diuretics	Antihistamines	Resorcinol
	Banthine	Nitrites
	4. Cardiac failure	

This data collected from various sources in 1971 by J. D. Davidson, M.D., Nuclear Medicine Section, Department of Radiology, Duke University Medical Center, Durham, N.C.
    ACTH = adrenocorticotropic hormone; PASA = paraaminosalicylic acid; PABA = para-aminobenzoic acid.

Radioactive Thyroid Uptake. Thyroid uptake of radioactive tracers is based on the concept of trapping and retention of iodine by the thyroid gland. The thyroid gland utilizes radioactive tracers in the same fashion as it does iodine obtained from dietary sources. The percentage of tracer concentrated within the thyroid gland is, therefore, inversely proportional to the iodine obtained from dietary sources.

Conditions relating to an accurate determination of thyroid activity include a normal iodide pool within the body (i.e., if the pool is increased abnormally, as from iodide obtained from roentgenographic contrast material, the amount of tracer trapped by the thyroid gland will be reduced, resulting in a falsely low determination of thyroid activity); an acceptable level of renal function; and lack of interference from medications (refer to Table 12-1).

The examination is performed by giving the patient a predetermined amount of ^{131}I, usually in the form of a capsule. The thyroid area is then counted at 4- and 24-hour periods, with the amount of activity retained in the thyroid expressed as a percentage of the dose administered. The 4-hour uptake is useful to reveal some states of hyperthyroidism, and the 24-hour uptake is generally necessary to demonstrate hypothyroidism.

The thyroid uptake will separate hyperthyroidism from the normal state with a 90 percent accuracy. In equivocal cases, a thyroid suppression test may be obtained by administering 75 to 150 mg of T_3 for three to seven days following a thyroid uptake. In normal patients the thyroid uptake will be suppressed more than 30 percent of the base value; no appreciable effect will be seen in patients with hyperthyroidism.

Differentiation between primary and secondary hypothyroidism can be determined by administering TSH, the pituitary hormone, in the amount of 10 units intramuscularly for three days. A return to normal value would indicate hypopituitary disease; no change would be indicative of primary thyroid failure. This thyroid-stimulatory test is about 70 percent accurate.

T_3 Uptake Tests. A T_3 uptake test is performed on patient serum (in vitro); thus, the patient receives no radiation. As with ^{131}I uptake, there must be a normal protein pool and no medicinal interference with thyroid binding. Table 12-2 lists common conditions and medications causing changes in T_3 uptake tests.

The T_3 test is an indirect measurement of the binding rate of thyroxine or triiodothyronine to plasma proteins. Radioactive T_3 is added to serum in the presence of a secondary binding site (red blood cells or ion exchange resin). After incubation, the secondary site is removed. From the amount of radioactive T_3 remaining in the patient's serum, the percentage saturation of binding sites is determined. Normal values vary from laboratory to laboratory, but acceptable base lines are 28 to 35 percent for the resin; a value above these levels indicates hyperthyroidism and below, hypothyroidism. As with the ^{131}I uptake, several drug compounds interfere with the results of the examination. These are noted in Table 12-2.

Some of the newer in vitro examinations include the T_4 resin test, which

Table 12-2

Factors Other Than Inherent Thyroid Functional Status Which Affect T_3 and T_4 Test Results

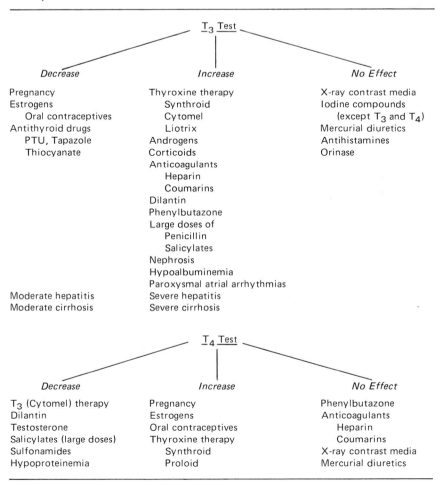

T_3 Test		
Decrease	*Increase*	*No Effect*
Pregnancy	Thyroxine therapy	X-ray contrast media
Estrogens	Synthroid	Iodine compounds
Oral contraceptives	Cytomel	(except T_3 and T_4)
Antithyroid drugs	Liotrix	Mercurial diuretics
PTU, Tapazole	Androgens	Antihistamines
Thiocyanate	Corticoids	Orinase
	Anticoagulants	
	Heparin	
	Coumarins	
	Dilantin	
	Phenylbutazone	
	Large doses of	
	Penicillin	
	Salicylates	
	Nephrosis	
	Hypoalbuminemia	
	Paroxysmal atrial arrhythmias	
Moderate hepatitis	Severe hepatitis	
Moderate cirrhosis	Severe cirrhosis	

T_4 Test		
Decrease	*Increase*	*No Effect*
T_3 (Cytomel) therapy	Pregnancy	Phenylbutazone
Dilantin	Estrogens	Anticoagulants
Testosterone	Oral contraceptives	Heparin
Salicylates (large doses)	Thyroxine therapy	Coumarins
Sulfonamides	Synthroid	X-ray contrast media
Hypoproteinemia	Proloid	Mercurial diuretics

This data collected from various sources in 1971 by J. D. Davidson, M.D., Nuclear Medicine Section, Department of Radiology, Duke University Medical Center, Durham, N.C.

measures total serum thyroxine. Column T_3 or T_4 studies are performed by pouring a diluted serum sample through a resin column and counting the collected eluate. Column T_3 or T_4 examinations are generally quicker, simpler, and as accurate as other T_3 resin tests.

Radioactive T_3 and T_4 examinations are used to evaluate the progress of treatment of hypothyroid or hyperthyroid states. Unlike the protein-bound iodine (PBD) or ^{131}I uptake tests, they are not appreciably affected by extraneous iodine and may be useful in detecting diseases not yet clinically manifested. One should be reminded that treatment of thyroid conditions must be based on the clinical state of the patient rather than on laboratory tests.

Thyroid Scanning. As has been noted before, the thyroid gland traps iodine and retains it until release mechanisms permit thyroid hormones to enter the bloodstream. If while performing a ^{131}I uptake one gives the patient an additional amount of tracer (30 to 100 μCi), a scan of the thyroid can be obtained at the same time the 24-hour uptake is determined. Scans may be helpful in evaluating thyroid nodules, carcinoma, substernal extension of the thyroid gland, and the size and shape of the thyroid gland. Care should be taken that scans are not obtained unnecessarily, with resultant excessive radiation to the patient.

The normal thyroid gland is extremely variable in size and shape. It is unusual to see symmetrical lobes, and an isthmus may not be demonstrated.

In evaluating for thyroid nodules, activity within the nodule is a determining factor. Hyperfunctioning nodules or lobes will have an increased area of activity as compared to normal tissue, while hypofunctioning areas will have decreased activity. At the same time the scan is performed, the patient's neck is palpated; and any palpable nodules are recorded on the "dot," or paper scan. Palpation of the thyroid is critical in determining hypoactivity or hyperactivity. Mislocation of a nodule may result in its being classified as hypoactive, whereas exact localization may cause a correct classification as normal activity. Evaluation of thyroid nodules is probably the most important use of thyroid scans.

Hyperfunctioning nodules are generally classified as *hot,* and *cold* nodules denote areas of hypofunction. Solitary cold nodules are generally believed to be surgical lesions since there is a reported increased incidence (10 to 25 percent) of carcinoma in these areas.

All in all, radioactive thyroid tests are good indicators of thyroid activity. The T_3 study is considered the safest and most accurate examination as compared to the PBI or ^{131}I uptake. The PBI has generally been replaced by radioactive thyroid tests. Figures 12-11 through 12-13 are representative examples of thyroid scanning.

SPECIAL EXAMINATIONS PERFORMED
IN NUCLEAR MEDICINE LABORATORIES

Schilling Test. A Schilling test is an examination useful in the determination of the levels of vitamin B_{12} (cyanocobalamin) within the body system. Deficiency of vitamin B_{12} results in a macrocytic anemia (pernicious anemia), and prolonged deficiency may result in neural degeneration. Vitamin B_{12} combines with an

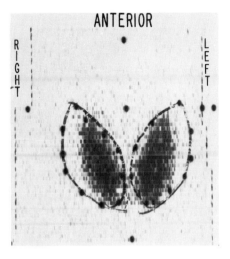

Fig. 12-11.
Normal thyroid scan. The lobes are equal in size and configuration. The outline was made by palpating the gland and marking the scan.

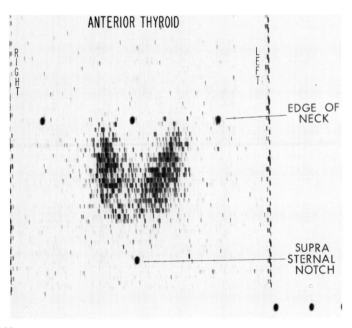

Fig. 12-12.
Thyroid scan with patchy uptake in a patient with hypothyroidism.

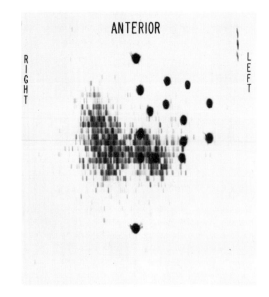

Fig. 12-13.
Large "cold" nodule in left lobe of thyroid gland shown to be a colloid cyst at surgery.

intrinsic factor produced in the stomach and is absorbed in the distal small bowel. Deficiency of vitamin B_{12} may be due to the body's inability to absorb the vitamin because of the absence of the intrinsic factor, which may be due either to a lack of synthesis or activation of the factor by the gastric mucosa. The deficiency may be due to the lack of gastric mucosa, itself, i.e., total gastrectomy; or it may be caused by a lack of absorption secondary to other gastrointestinal diseases, such as sprue or regional enteritis. In the presence of abnormal bacterial flora within the gastrointestinal tract, there may be malabsorption of the vitamin due to destruction or deactivation of the vitamin or its intrinsic factor.

A Schilling test is performed by giving the patient Co 57 cyanocobalamin orally together with 1,000 μg units of B_{12} intramuscularly in order to saturate B_{12}-binding sites and flush this large excess out in the urine. Since the binding sites are saturated, if oral B_{12} labeled with Co 57 is normally absorbed, it is largely excreted in the urine. The total urine output is then collected over a 48-hour period. If the results are not within normal range ($>$ 7 percent), the study is repeated with the addition of the intrinsic factor. Another collection of urine over a 24-hour period is then examined; and if the patient has pernicious anemia or a subtotal gastrectomy, the urine value should be normal. Care must be taken that there is no background radiation which could interfere with the test; and there must be a complete collection of the urine sample, since the loss of a small volume of urine may produce abnormal results.

If the examination is still abnormal after the study with the intrinsic factor, the patient may be given a broad-spectrum antibiotic over a period of one week to reduce any abnormal gastrointestinal bacterial flora and the examination may be performed again. If the abnormal bacterial flora have been replaced by normal flora, the examination will, therefore, be normal. If the examination still shows a low value, it can be presumed that the malabsorption is due to other problems such as sprue or regional enteritis.

Vitamin B_{12} absorption thus is useful in the primary diagnosis of pernicious anemia and is also helpful in the diagnostic work-up of anemia associated with intestinal parasites, abnormal intestinal bacterial flora, diverticulosis of the colon and small bowel, regional enteritis, and so on. It is of greatest value in separating pernicious anemia from malabsorption problems.

Fat Absorption Studies. In order for the body to absorb a neutral fat (e.g., triolein) from the gastrointestinal tract, adequate pancreatic enzymes, biliary function, and normal gastrointestinal absorption must be present. With fatty acids (e.g., oleic acid), pancreatic enzymatic action is not required and only gastrointestinal absorption and adequate biliary function are necessary. Fat absorption studies are therefore useful in the evaluation of patients with malabsorption or pancreatic disease. By giving the patient triolein I 131 or oleic acid I 131, one can determine the amount of fat absorbed into the blood and that amount which is excreted in the feces. After oral administration of the ^{131}I-labeled tracer, blood samples are obtained over a period of time and standardized according to blood volume. An average normal result is 15 percent absorbed. Urine-free stool collections are also gathered over a 72-hour period, and the iodinated fat excreted is calculated. An average result is approximately 1 percent excreted. It should be reemphasized that the stools must be free of radioactive-contaminated urine in order to have an accurate fecal excretion level.

If the triolein test is performed first and is normal, the test is essentially complete because in order to have normal absorption there must be adequate gastrointestinal absorption, adequate pancreatic enzymes, and adequate biliary function. If the test is abnormal, it is repeated using tagged oleic acid. If at this time the test is normal, the deficiency must be associated with pancreatic enzymatic insufficiency. If both tests are abnormal, malabsorption would be favored over some other etiology. Radioactive examinations of this type are generally not as sensitive as chemical determinations but do serve as good screening tests.

Protein Loss from the Gastrointestinal Tract. Protein enteropathy may occur from a number of diseases of the gastrointestinal tract. Radioactive tracers may be given to the patient intravenously; and the amount lost in the stools over a given time, usually 96 hours, is measured and may indicate a useful screening or confirmation procedure for the gastrointestinal enteropathy. A number of pathological entities are associated with gastrointestinal loss of protein, such as tumors of the gastrointestinal tract, infections, anatomical abnormalities such as stenoses and diverticuloses, and the nonspecific inflammatory diseases such as gastritis, Menetrier's disease, sprue, regional enteritis, and ulcerative colitis. Non-gastrointestinal diseases include constrictive pericarditis, thrombosis of the inferior vena cava, nephrotic syndrome, and the abnormal gamma globulinemias.

The study is performed by giving the patient serum albumin Cr 51 or chloride Cr 51 intravenously, and urine-free stools are collected for 96 hours. Less than 1 percent of the injected chromium 51 should be recovered in the stools of a normal patient. Values greater than 1 percent indicate malabsorption of the labeled protein. This is a relatively simple procedure done in nuclear medicine.

Blood Volumes. One of the simplest procedures done in nuclear medicine is the determination of blood volumes. The study is based on the dilution principle. A known quantity of human serum albumin I 131 is given intravenously. Blood samples are drawn at a later time, usually in ten or fifteen minutes, and the dilution is compared against the standard. By the dilution factor technique one can estimate the dilution of the tracer within the blood or plasma and relate it to the standard. This method is not as accurate as the red cell blood volume study but is much easier to perform and can be done much more rapidly.

The blood volume determinations performed using labeled red blood cells require several hours to perform, since the plasma volume and red cell mass must both be calculated. Blood is withdrawn from the patient and the red cells are tagged with chromium 51 and reinjected into the patient, with blood volume estimated by the dilution technique. It may require several hours to tag the red cells with chromium 51, but true blood volume determination is more accurate than that obtained from the test performed with the ^{131}I-labeled serum albumin dilution technique.

Other Examinations. Red cell survival time can be calculated by withdrawing red cells from the patient and labeling them with chromium 51. Blood samples are then drawn daily over a period of two to three weeks and the rate of decreasing tracer activity plotted on semilog paper, with the mean normal chromium 51 survival time being approximately 28 days. The same technique may be used for spleen scanning.

Again by withdrawing the patient's red cells, tagging them with chromium 51, and then reinjecting them into the patient, one can determine the amount of sequestration of the red cells by the spleen. This may be done in conjunction with the red cell survival study. Counts over the liver, spleen, and heart are made and compared to each other. The basic factor is that the counts over the spleen should be twice what they are over the liver.

Iron studies are useful in determining or evaluating a number of hematological disorders. The plasma iron clearance is useful in differentiating different types of anemias. If ^{59}Fe-labeled ferrous citrate is given to the patient intravenously and samples of plasma are made and plotted against time on log paper, the time required for ^{59}Fe counts to decline 50 percent is normally one to two hours. In such conditions as polycythemia, hemolytic anemia, and iron-deficiency anemia, the time required to remove one-half the tracer is shortened. However, in other abnormalities such as hypoplastic anemia and myelofibrosis, it is prolonged. By obtaining the plasma iron value determined chemically and utilizing the plasma volume and the half-time of clearing of the iron-labeled citrate, the plasma iron turnover rate can be calculated. At the same time, the utilization of the iron into circulating red cells can also be calculated.

READING LIST

General

Blahd, W. H. (Ed.). *Nuclear Medicine.* New York: Blakiston Div., McGraw-Hill, 1965.
Gottschalk, A., and Beck, R. N. *Fundamental Problems in Scanning.* Springfield, Ill.: Thomas, 1968.
Maynard, C. D. *Clinical Nuclear Medicine.* Philadelphia: Lea & Febiger, 1969.
Silver, S. *Radioactive Nuclides in Medicine and Biology,* 3d ed. Philadelphia: Lea & Febiger, 1968.
Wagner, H. N., Jr. (Ed.). *Principles of Nuclear Medicine.* Philadelphia: Saunders, 1968.
Wang, Y. *Clinical Radioisotope Scanning.* Springfield, Ill.: Thomas, 1967.

Specific

DeLand, F. H., and Wagner, H. N., Jr. *Atlas of Nuclear Medicine.* Philadelphia: Saunders, 1969.
Physicians' Desk Reference for Radiology and Nuclear Medicine. Oradell, N.J.: Medical Economics, Inc., 1971.

Special Procedures in Radiology 13

UNTIL A FEW DECADES AGO, special procedures in radiology included any-thing other than routine roentgenographic procedures. Hence, in some depart-ments gallbladder examinations, upper gastrointestinal series, and barium enemas were considered special procedures to be performed as time would allow. As roentgenographic techniques have become more sophisticated, one speaks of special procedures to include such things as angiography, pneumoencephalog-raphy, lymphangiography, mammography, and diagnostic ultrasound. A brief description of these procedures is included to provide the student a better con-cept of the role the radiologist plays in the care of patients.

Lymphangiography. Lymphangiography is a procedure in which the lymph node channels are opacified to detect the presence of disease. One of the more com-mon uses of lymphangiography is to evaluate the abdominal lymph node chains for staging of lymphoma and for evaluation of lymphedema. Through injection of the lymph channels in the hands, the axillary and supraclavicular nodes may be identified and evaluated. By injecting the lymph channels in the feet, the inguinal, iliac, paraaortic, and occasionally the supraclavicular nodes may be inspected.

The procedure is performed by aseptically injecting a dye (for example, Evans blue) that has been diluted with procaine topical anesthetic into the webs of the second and third toes or fingers. The dye is taken up by the lymph and trans-ported to the lymph vessels. After allowing sufficient time for enough dye to be visualized in the lymph channels (about ten minutes), the lymph vessel is dissected free and then cannulated with a No. 29 or 30 lymphangiographic needle. Contrast material is then injected under pressure with the aid of lymph-angiographic pumps.

After injection of the contrast media is completed, films of the extremity and lymph node chains are obtained. These films show early filling of the lymph nodes and vessels and are valuable primarily for that purpose. Twenty-four hours later the lymph nodes normally have become filled with the contrast material, and films of the lymph node chains are again obtained. The excess of contrast material flows into the thoracic duct and is deposited as microemboli in the lungs, where it gradually disappears.

Lymphangiography may require two or three hours to perform. In some patients it is extremely difficult to cannulate a lymph channel; and, needless to say, the radiologist must have a steady hand and a relaxed, cooperative patient in order to have a successful end to the procedure. Since the lymphangiographic needles may be precariously placed, it is extremely important that the patient not move his feet (or hands) so as to dislodge the needles. Some radiologists have referred to this procedure as "starting an IV on a fly."

As with any other examination using contrast material, contraindications include a medical history of an allergic or adverse reaction to iodine or iodine-containing drugs. In addition, previous radiation to the lungs and chronic pulmonary disease with pulmonary function less than 70 percent of normal are generally contraindications. Previous irradiation of lymph node chains should make the radiologist approach the examination with caution, since contrast material may be dumped directly into the lungs without benefit of filtration by the lymph nodes.

The incision made for a lymphangiogram should receive the same quality of care as any other surgical incision. If the area is neglected, stitch abscesses may occur and present a problem in healing.

Normal lymph nodes present a regular, uniform opacity (Fig. 13-1). Lymphomatous nodes are foamy in appearance and usually are enlarged (Fig. 13-2). Metastatic tumor shows replacement or filling defects in the peripheral sinusoids of the lymph glands. In granulomatous disease, the lymph nodes are enlarged; but the internal architecture and peripheral sinusoids are preserved. Some lymph nodes may be completely replaced by tumor and not opacified. Displacement of the lymph node chain more than 2.5 cm lateral to the vertebral bodies or 3.0 cm anteriorly is pathological, even if the lymph nodes themselves appear normal.

Roentgenograms of inguinal lymph nodes should be interpreted with caution. Chronic, minute inflammatory lesions, particularly in the feet, create chronic inflammatory changes in the inguinal nodes draining the area. It is therefore common to see enlarged inguinal nodes in the absence of other enlarged nodes. The lymph nodes in the region of the hilum of the left kidney drain the skin area surrounding the scrotum and may also become enlarged, with no other abnormalities seen in the lymph node chains.

Lymphangiography is also used in evaluation of edema of the extremities. In lymphedema, there may be absent or hypoplastic lymph trunks, with varicosities even seen. The role of lymphangiography is to determine whether or not the lymphatic system is obstructed. If the lymphatic system is open, it is suggested that the cause of lymphedema may be venous rather than actually lymphatic in nature.

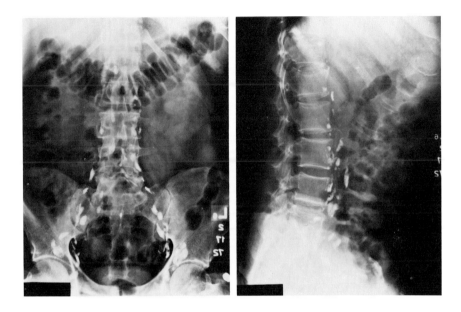

Fig. 13-1.
Normal lymphangiogram. The opacified lymph nodes are normal in size, show no
displacement, and have a normal internal architecture.

Diagnostic Ultrasound. During World War I, SONAR (sound ranging and detection) was introduced by the British to help combat the catastrophic sinkings of
surface vessels by German submarines in the North Atlantic Ocean. This technique was perfected in World War II and is widely used by industry in this
country to detect flaws in metals, cloths, and so on. From a specialized use of
reflected sound in warfare and industry, sonar has entered the medical field and
is fast becoming a major diagnostic device. Lack of major physical and biological
effects has enhanced its use, particularly in this day of greater cognizance of
radiation hazards and safety.

By definition, ultrasound is sound above the frequency of 16,000 cycles per
second, which is higher than the human ear can detect. The frequency most
commonly used in ultrasound for diagnosis varies from approximately 60 kilo-
cycles to 10 megacycles.

Only a few basic principles of diagnostic ultrasound need to be understood
in order to obtain a working knowledge of the clinical application of sonar
devices.

The process of sound propagation is quite similar to the game of billiards. If
a cue ball strikes a lead ball in the rack of billiard balls, the energy is transferred
from the cue ball to each ball in the rack until all billiard balls have absorbed

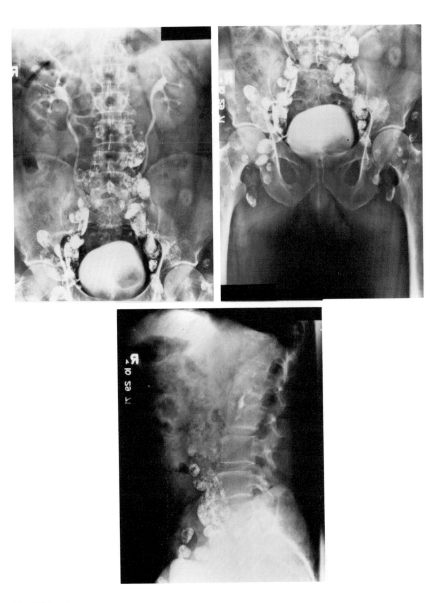

Fig. 13-2.
Lymphangiogram in Hodgkin's disease. Notice the enlarged, foamy lymph nodes displacing the ureters.

energy. The same thing happens in sound propagation. The sound wave is mechanically produced and directed toward an object. As the wave goes forward, it mechanically compresses air, fluid, or tissue immediately in front of it; and the secondary wave passes its energy on to the next area, and so forth. This is also quite analogous to tossing a stone in a smooth pond and watching the ripples going forth in a seemingly never-ending fashion from the point of impaction of the stone with the water. Such things as this occur in diagnostic ultrasound except that the oscillations produced are in a much higher frequency than imaginable in the analogies of the billiard ball or pond.

Sound waves are attenuated by the media into which they pass. Attenuation is affected both by the density of the media and the frequency of the sound wave propagated. Generally speaking, the greater the density, the further the sound will be propagated.

When two different substances with different densities are adjoined, the boundary between these two substances is known as an *interface.* For all practical purposes, there is always some reflection of energy from interfaces in the human body, and these interfaces are what one records and interprets in ultrasonography.

The most common use of diagnostic ultrasound is for the localization of the midline of the brain (Fig. 13-3). In this application the sound wave is passed through the skull and into the brain perpendicular to the falx and then bounced back to the receiving device; and the midline of the brain is recorded as a blip on the oscilloscope. By recording the sound waves from one side and then from the other side, the midline of the brain should always be in the same area. Ultrasound is quite diagnostic and requires only a few minutes to perform. It is

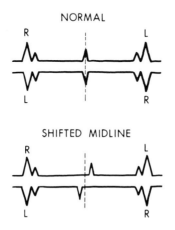

NORMAL

SHIFTED MIDLINE

Fig. 13-3.
Schematic depiction of (top) normal echoencephalogram; (bottom) shift of the midline.

particularly useful in emergency room settings in which a patient may be suspected of having a possible subdural hematoma. If there is a detectable space-occupying lesion within one side of the brain and not the other, there is a shift of the midline of the brain identified by a separation of blips from the right-to-left and left-to-right recordings.

Other applications of ultrasonography include examination of the chest for pulmonary emboli or the detection of aortic aneurysms. A great deal of work has been done in examination of the heart valves and in the diagnosis of pericardial effusion. The diagnostic ultrasound unit is a splendid method of following movement of cardiac valves after surgery.

The value of diagnostic ultrasound in obstetrics has been well recorded. There has been reported a 90 percent accuracy in determining the location of the placenta. Also, a monograph has been published in which the biparietal diameter of the fetal skull is recorded from a scanning laminograph and the fetal age closely approximated. The size of the uterus can also be approximated.

One of the most interesting uses of diagnostic ultrasound devices is in the evaluation of solid versus cystic lesions. In the presence of a cystic lesion, clear interfaces between the liquid of the cyst and the solid material of the wall can be demonstrated with ultrasound. This is quite useful in scanning kidney lesions in which one would like to differentiate between a solid tumor and a benign renal cyst.

Myelography. Myelography is the examination of the spinal canal performed by injecting a contrast material into the subarachnoid space by means of a lumbar puncture. As noted in Chapter 3, Pantopaque is most commonly used for this procedure. Since this drug is heavier than spinal fluid, it does not mix with the fluid but sinks to the dependent portion of the subarachnoid space. Following injection of the contrast material, the patient is positioned on a fluoroscopic table with the table tilted until the area in question is covered with the contrast material.

Indications for myelography are to evaluate degeneration of the spinal cord and to delineate suspicious or suspected mass lesions such as tumors or herniated intervertebral disks. Myelography is also used to locate spinal lesions when the neurological examination has not been definitive.

Mass lesions are generally described as extradural, intradural extramedullary, and intradural intramedullary. Extradural lesions are those in which the spinal cord is displaced away from its bony confines. Such conditions as intervertebral disk protrusions and metastatic tumors produce this type of defect. Intradural extramedullary lesions, usually neurofibromas or meningiomas, enlarge the cord within the confines of the spinal column and displace it to one side. Intradural intramedullary lesions produce fusiform expansion of the cord uniformly within the spinal canal and are usually ependymomas, astrocytomas, or syringomyelia.

By the nature of myelography an amount of spinal fluid is lost, and after the procedure the patient should have fluid forced and remain flat in bed to alleviate the headache usually associated with such a procedure. Myelography is not performed on those patients with suspected increase in intracranial pressure, since loss of the spinal fluid may precipitate herniation of the pons into the spinal canal. Figure 13-4 demonstrates some myelographic findings.

Mammography. Mammography is an x-ray examination of the breast (Fig. 13-5). This is a technique developed over the last few years in which extremely low kilovoltage (25 to 30 kv) and high milliamperage (300 to 1,500) are used to obtain the ultimate in roentgenographic contrast. Particular care is taken that the roentgenographic exposures are exact and that the x-ray films are optimally processed.

Mammography is quite useful in screening breasts for tumors and evaluating lumps within the breasts. Egan has reported over 90 percent accuracy in differentiating benign from malignant lesions, and lesions as small as a few millimeters have been demonstrated.

Roentgenographically, malignant tumors such as scirrhous carcinomas may show an irregular, spiculated border; whereas the papillary type of carcinoma may be well circumscribed. Fine, spiculated calcification is seen in over a third of the malignant tumors. Other signs include increased vascularity (veins) and thickening of the skin.

Benign lesions usually present as homogeneous densities within well-circumscribed borders. Calcification may be present, particularly in fibroadenomas; but the calcification is coarse rather than the fine, sandlike calcification seen in malignant tumors.

Angiography. Angiography is the procedure in which water-soluble contrast material is injected into a vessel. Phlebography is the same process except that the contrast material is injected into a vein. Arteriograms are roentgenograms of opacified arteries obtained during the angiographic procedure, and phlebograms are films of opacified veins. Selective angiograms are obtained by selectively catheterizing and injecting specific veins or arteries.

Approach or entrance into a vessel is by one of three different methods; by performing a cut-down on the vessel, by a percutaneous puncture, or by a percutaneous puncture with catheter insertion. The vascular radiologist may select any one of the three, depending upon the clinical situation of the patient and the information the radiologist wishes to obtain from the procedure.

As the term *percutaneous* implies, percutaneous arteriography is a procedure in which contrast material is injected into a vessel without the use of a surgical cut-down or exposure of the vessel. The procedure is performed by injecting the soft tissues surrounding a vessel with a topical anesthetic (such as lidocaine) in an aseptic manner. After suitable anesthesia is obtained, a small nick is made in the skin over the vessel. While the vessel is palpated with one hand, a No. 18

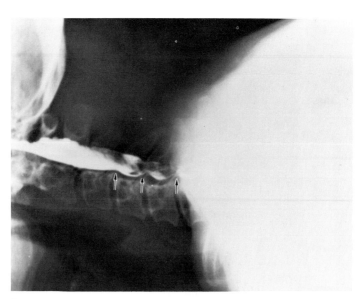

A

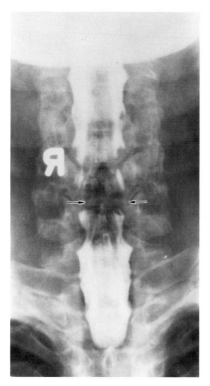

B

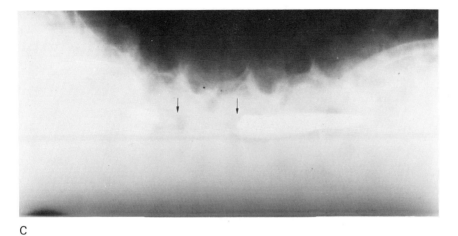

C

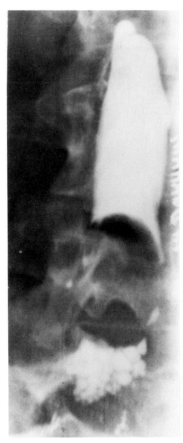

D

Fig. 13-4.

Myelography. (A, B) Spondylosis of the cervical spine creating defects in the Pantopaque column. (C, D) Intradural intramedullary defect of the lumber spinal column.

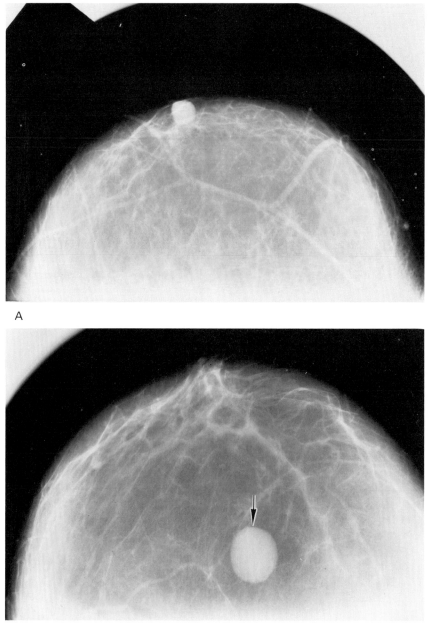

A

B

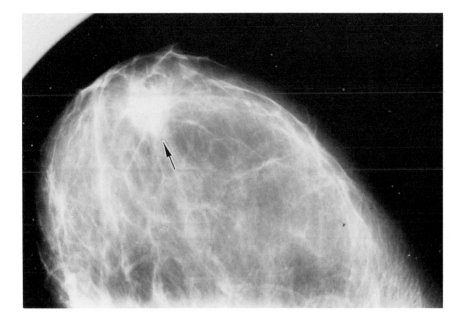

C

Fig. 13-5.
  Mammography. (A) Normal postmenopausal breast, cephalocaudad projection.
(B) Benign cyst. (C) Scirrhous carcinoma. Notice the irregularity of this lesion as com-
pared to that in (B).

needle with an obturator is passed through both walls of the vessel. The obturator is removed from the needle, and a slight downward pressure is exerted on
the hub as it is slowly withdrawn. As the needle passes through the posterior
wall of the vessel, it slips into the vascular lumen and blood flow is obtained.
(In phlebography the same process is used except that a syringe is applied to the
hub of the needle to obtain a slight negative pressure.) After blood flow is obtained, the obturator is replaced and the needle slowly advanced within the
vessel until the hub rests against the skin. An injection of the contrast material
can then be made.
  With the catheter technique, a different type of needle is used — one containing a sheath around the needle — and the puncture is made in the same fashion.
In some situations contrast material can be injected directly through the needle
or through the nylon sheath. If a catheter is to be inserted, the needle is withdrawn, leaving behind the sheath which serves as a channel through which to
insert a guide wire. With maintenance of pressure on the nylon sheath to prevent bleeding, the guide wire is advanced through the sheath until it is in its
proper location. The tip of the guide wire is quite flexible so as to prevent

dissection of the intima of the vessel or dislodging of arteriosclerotic plaques from the intima of the vessel.

After the guide wire is in a suitable location, the needle sheath is removed and a catheter inserted over the guide wire and advanced to its proper location. The guide wire is then removed, and the catheter is connected to a syringe or other apparatus for continuous effusion so as to prevent air bubbles from entering the arterial system. Small volumes of contrast material are sporadically injected until the catheter tip is in its exact, proper location. The patient is then centered over the film changer or cine unit, and a volume of contrast material is injected while x-ray exposures are made. With modern catheters and techniques available, almost any vessel in the body can be reached and opacified.

Approach to vessels may be through the femoral, brachial, axillary, carotid, or, occasionally, the vertebral arteries or companion veins. Most catheter approaches are through the axillary or femoral routes, and direct arterial punctures are either through the brachial or carotid pathways. Retrograde brachial arteriograms (BAG) are used to opacify the great vessels arising from the aortic arch. Carotid arteriograms (CAG) are used to visualize the carotid arteries and intracranial vessels. From the axillary and femoral approaches, almost any vessel can be cannulated and opacified.

Angiography may also be performed, particularly in operating rooms, in which the vessel in question is exposed surgically and a needle is inserted, with contrast material then injected.

Angiography (phlebography) (Fig. 13-6) is used to evaluate patency or competency of vessels following trauma; to visualize vascular supply and thus possible diagnosis of mass lesions; to depict abnormal vasculature arising from tumors and thus help differentiate benign from malignant conditions; to provide surgical maps for physicians; to evaluate arteriosclerotic changes in vessels; to study congenital and acquired heart disease; to delineate competency of peripheral veins; and to investigate a host of other entities. Anticancer drugs are also selectively injected into vessels feeding tumors. Analytic blood samples may be obtained from selected arteries or veins.

The complications seen from angiography are usually secondary to the procedure. Blood clots form readily on the catheter and may be dislocated and produce vascular infarction. Injections may be made inadvertently into the walls of the vessel and create a dissection or occlusion. A vessel may be ruptured or torn, leading to hemorrhage. Arteriosclerotic plaques may be knocked loose from the vessel wall and form emboli. Reactions may also occur to the contrast material, as can happen in any other procedure.

Portophlebography. The portal venous system may be visualized by any one of three methods: (1) injection of contrast material into the portal system may be performed at the time of surgical exploration of the abdomen; (2) large volumes of contrast material may be simultaneously injected into the celiac axis and

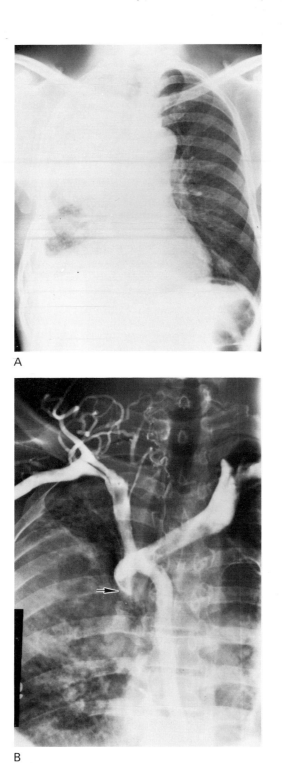

A

B

Figure 13-6

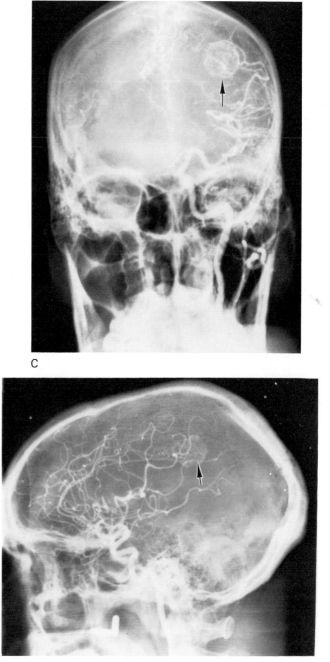

C

D

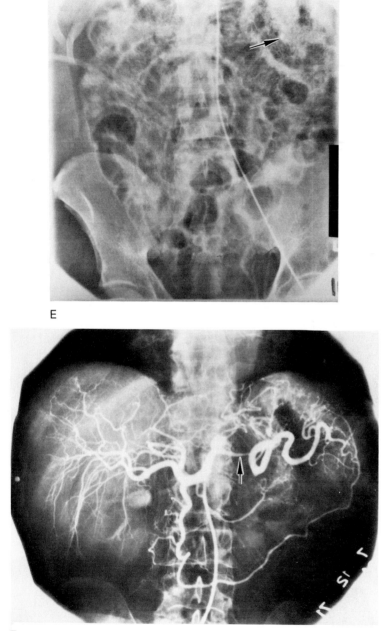

E

F

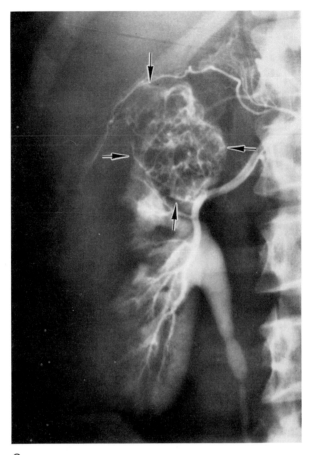

G

Fig. 13-6.
Uses of arteriography and phlebography. (A, B) Carcinoma of the lung occluding the superior vena cava. (C, D) Cerebral arteriogram demonstrating metastatic tumor to the brain. (E) Selective superior mesenteric arteriogram demonstrating a bleeding site. (F) Selective splenic artery injection demonstrating encasement of the splenic artery by pancreatic carcinoma. (G) Renal arteriogram demonstrating hypernephroma.

superior mesenteric arteries with transcapillary visualization of the portal system; (3) contrast material may be injected percutaneously into the splenic pulp with resultant visualization of the splenic veins and portal system (Fig. 13-7).

In addition to the normal contraindications to doing a special procedure, such as a previous history of allergy to the contrast material, special contraindications for these types of studies should also be noted. Before performing a percutaneous splenoportogram, the patient must have normal bleeding, clotting, and prothrombin times and normal platelet counts. There should be no ascites, since in this condition the spleen is quite movable and the patient may have increased bleeding following the procedure due to lack of fixation of the spleen. There must be adequate liver or renal function to excrete the contrast material. During this procedure there is usually some loss of blood, but rarely does the patient need a transfusion.

The indications for doing such procedures are to provide a surgical map of the vascular system, to evaluate portal hypertension and the presence of varices, to evaluate occlusion or thrombosis of the portal system, and to depict colateral

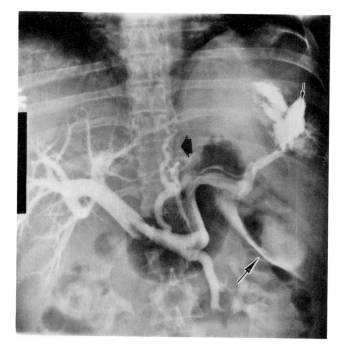

Fig. 13-7.
    Splenoportogram. Notice the stain in the splenic pulp and extravasation of the contrast material around the splenic capsule. Esophageal varices are seen at solid arrow.

blood flow. Following the procedure the patient should have bed rest and forced fluids. Vital signs and hematocrit should be followed to detect blood loss.

Percutaneous Cholangiography. As noted in Chapter 7, percutaneous cholangiography (Fig. 13-8) is a procedure in which a long needle is inserted aseptically through the anesthetized skin and the biliary tree punctured. Bile is withdrawn and partially replaced with a water-soluble contrast medium, and the biliary tree is examined. The indication for such a procedure is obstructive jaundice associated with a rising serum bilirubin.

The same bleeding precautions as noted under Portophlebography should be taken. In addition, an operating room should be immediately available with prearrangements made with the surgeon, since on occasion the patient may suffer uncontrollable bleeding from the hepatic vascular supply and thus need a laparotomy. Vital signs and hematocrit must be checked periodically after the procedure to elicit early signs of blood loss.

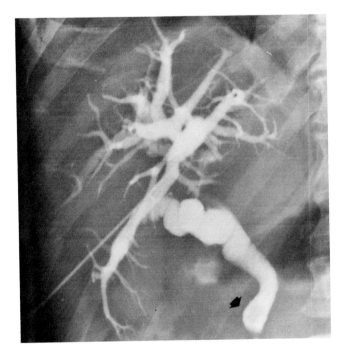

Fig. 13-8.
    Percutaneous cholangiogram. Large radiolucent stone demonstrated in the distal common duct.

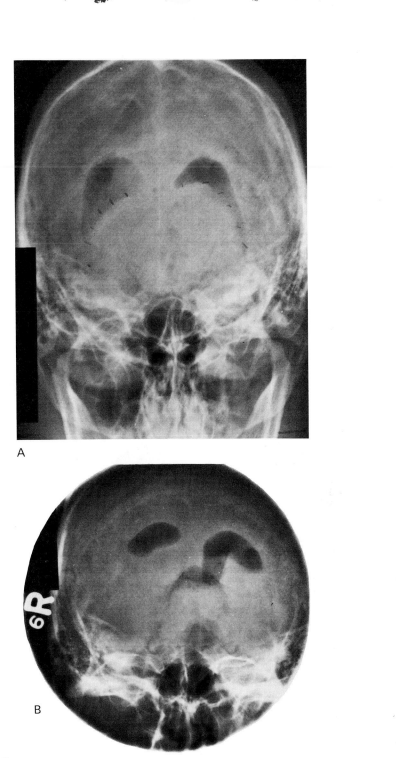

A

B

Figure 13-9

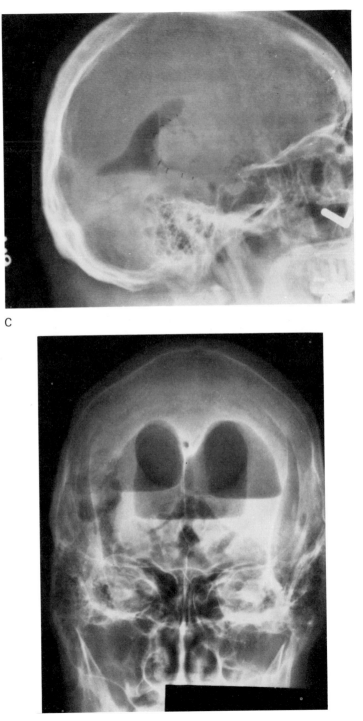

C

D

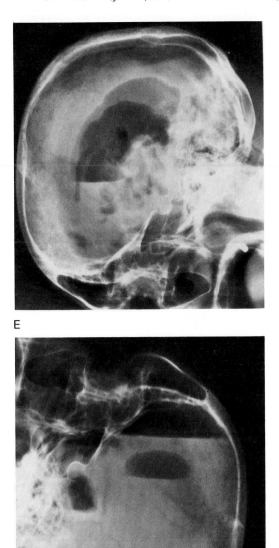

E

F

Fig. 13-9.

Pneumoencephalography. (A, B, C) Large hypothalamic tumor displacing ventricle. (D, E, F) Marked low-pressure hydrocephalus.

Pneumoencephalography. The injection of air through a lumbar puncture needle and subsequent migration of air into the ventricles of the brain, subarachnoid cisterns, and subarachnoid spaces of the brain is known as air encephalography or pneumoencephalography. Injection of air into the ventricular system through a burr hole in the skull is known as ventriculography.

Pneumoencephalography is performed by inserting a lumbar puncture needle into the lumbar subarachnoid space. Small increments of cerebrospinal fluid are withdrawn and replaced with air. The head is manipulated so as to allow the air to gravitate and outline a specific portion of the subarachnoid cisterns or ventricular system, and appropriate roentgenographic views of the skull are obtained.

The intracranial ventricular system and subarachnoid cisterns are sensitive indicators of displacement from their normal anatomical locations by intracranial mass lesions. Obstruction to the circulation or reabsorption of cerebrospinal fluid may also be shown. Flow of the cerebrospinal fluid is important, since dilatation of the ventricular system proximal to a site of obstruction usually indicates the point of obstruction. Increasing production of cerebrospinal fluid or obstruction to its flow may result in herniation of the cerebellar tonsils through the foramen magnum and compression of the upper spinal cord, which may lead to death. Figure 13-9 illustrates some pneumoencephalographic changes.

Patient preparation and care after the procedure are important. Normally the patient is sedated with some type of barbiturate and given atropine prior to the procedure. Analgesics are not used, since they may mask signs and symptoms of tonsillar herniation. The replacement of cerebrospinal fluid by air changes the physiological pressure system within the cranial vault and leads to rather severe headaches which may be accompanied by nausea and vomiting. Hydration, strict bed rest with the head flat, and analgesics are necessary after the procedure. Generally these symptoms will have subsided after 24 to 48 hours.

Other special procedures done by the radiologist include sinus tract injections, perirenal carbon dioxide insufflation, gynecography and hysterosalpingography, sialography, hypotonic duodenography, and peritoneal double-contrast examinations. The radiologist is a useful person to consult about different approaches to detection and diagnosis of disease processes.

READING LIST

Abrams, H. L. *Angiography,* 2d ed. Boston: Little, Brown, 1971.

Egan, R. L. *Mammography,* 2d ed. Springfield, Ill.: Thomas, 1972.

Grossman, C. C. (Ed.). *Diagnostic Ultrasound.* Philadelphia: Lippincott, 1966.

Schobinger, R. A., and Ruzicka, F. F., Jr. (Eds.). *Vascular Roentgenology.* New York: Macmillan, 1964.

Taveras, J. M., and Wood, E. H. *Diagnostic Neuroradiology.* Baltimore: Williams & Wilkins, 1964.

Wolfe, J. N. *Mammography.* Springfield, Ill.: Thomas, 1967.

Appendix: Bony Anatomy

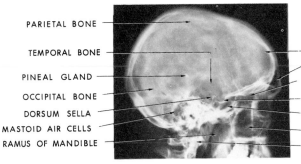

PARIETAL BONE

TEMPORAL BONE

PINEAL GLAND

OCCIPITAL BONE

DORSUM SELLA

MASTOID AIR CELLS

RAMUS OF MANDIBLE

FRONTAL BONE

FRONTAL SINUSES

ETHMOIDAL SINUSES

SELLA TURCICA

SPHENOID SINUSES

MAXILLARY SINUSES

ODONTOID

Fig. A-1.
Lateral view of the skull.

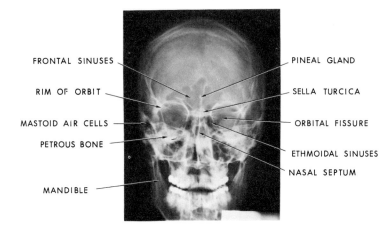

FRONTAL SINUSES

RIM OF ORBIT

MASTOID AIR CELLS

PETROUS BONE

MANDIBLE

PINEAL GLAND

SELLA TURCICA

ORBITAL FISSURE

ETHMOIDAL SINUSES

NASAL SEPTUM

Fig. A-2.
Posteroanterior view of the skull.

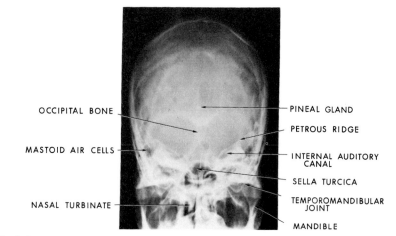

OCCIPITAL BONE   PINEAL GLAND

                                          PETROUS RIDGE

MASTOID AIR CELLS   INTERNAL AUDITORY
                                           CANAL

                                          SELLA TURCICA

NASAL TURBINATE   TEMPOROMANDIBULAR
                                           JOINT

                                          MANDIBLE

Fig. A-3.
Towne view of the skull.

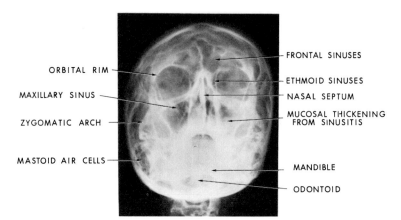

                                          FRONTAL SINUSES

ORBITAL RIM   ETHMOID SINUSES

MAXILLARY SINUS   NASAL SEPTUM

ZYGOMATIC ARCH   MUCOSAL THICKENING
                                           FROM SINUSITIS

MASTOID AIR CELLS   MANDIBLE

                                          ODONTOID

Fig. A-4.
Water's view of the skull.

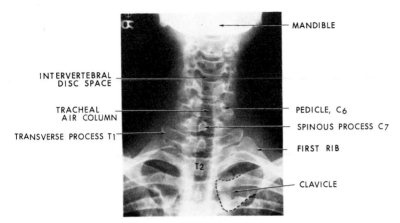

Fig. A-5.

Anteroposterior view of the cervical spine.

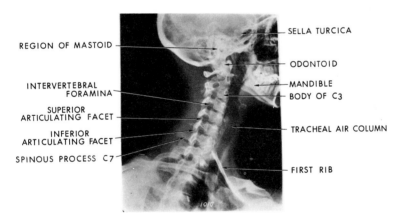

Fig. A-6.

Oblique view of the cervical spine.

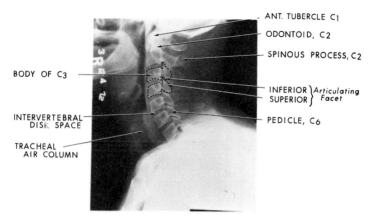

Fig. A-7.

Lateral view of the cervical spine.

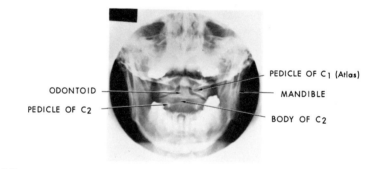

Fig. A-8.

Transoral view of odontoid.

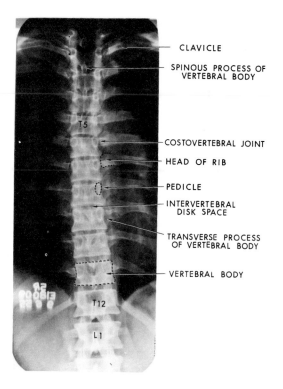

Fig. A-9.

Anteroposterior view of the thoracic spine.

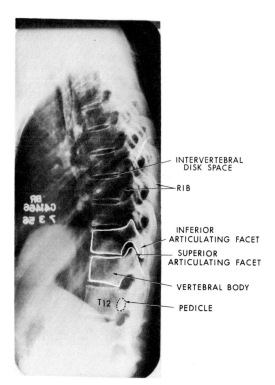

INTERVERTEBRAL
DISK SPACE

RIB

INFERIOR
ARTICULATING FACET

SUPERIOR
ARTICULATING FACET

VERTEBRAL BODY

PEDICLE

Fig. A-10.
Lateral view of the thoracic spine.

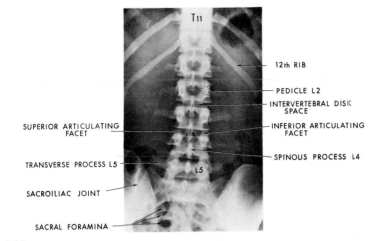

Fig. A-11.

Anteroposterior view of the lumbar spine.

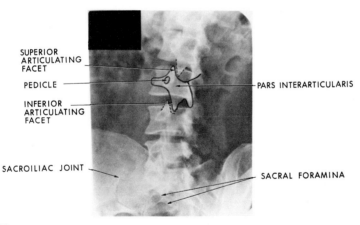

Fig. A-12.

Oblique view of the lumbar spine.

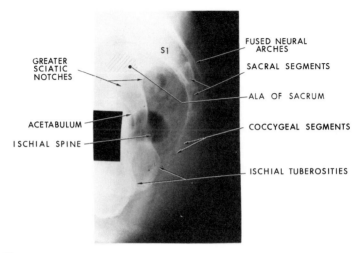

Fig. A-13.
Lateral view of the coccyx.

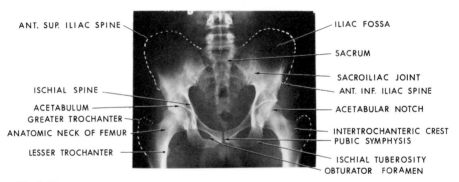

Fig. A-14.
Anteroposterior view of the pelvis.

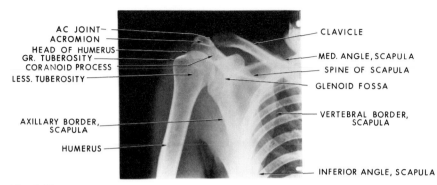

AC JOINT—
ACROMION
HEAD OF HUMERUS
GR. TUBEROSITY
CORANOID PROCESS
LESS. TUBEROSITY

CLAVICLE
MED. ANGLE, SCAPULA
SPINE OF SCAPULA
GLENOID FOSSA

AXILLARY BORDER,
SCAPULA

VERTEBRAL BORDER,
SCAPULA

HUMERUS

INFERIOR ANGLE, SCAPULA

Fig. A-15.
Anteroposterior view of the shoulder.

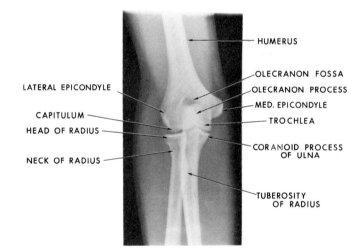

HUMERUS

LATERAL EPICONDYLE

OLECRANON FOSSA
OLECRANON PROCESS
MED. EPICONDYLE

CAPITULUM
HEAD OF RADIUS

TROCHLEA

NECK OF RADIUS

CORANOID PROCESS
OF ULNA

TUBEROSITY
OF RADIUS

Fig. A-16.
Anteroposterior view of the elbow.

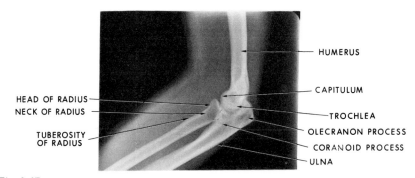

Fig. A-17.
Lateral view of the elbow.

HEAD OF RADIUS
NECK OF RADIUS
TUBEROSITY OF RADIUS
HUMERUS
CAPITULUM
TROCHLEA
OLECRANON PROCESS
CORANOID PROCESS
ULNA

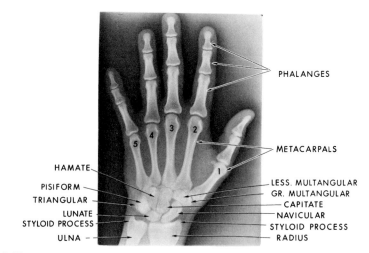

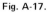

Fig. A-18.
Posteroanterior view of the hand.

PHALANGES
METACARPALS
HAMATE
PISIFORM
TRIANGULAR
LUNATE
STYLOID PROCESS
ULNA
LESS. MULTANGULAR
GR. MULTANGULAR
CAPITATE
NAVICULAR
STYLOID PROCESS
RADIUS

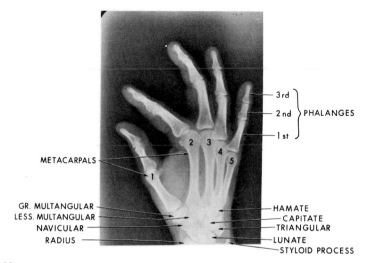

3rd
2nd } PHALANGES
1st

METACARPALS

GR. MULTANGULAR
LESS. MULTANGULAR
NAVICULAR
RADIUS

HAMATE
CAPITATE
TRIANGULAR
LUNATE
STYLOID PROCESS

Fig. A-19.
Oblique view of the hand.

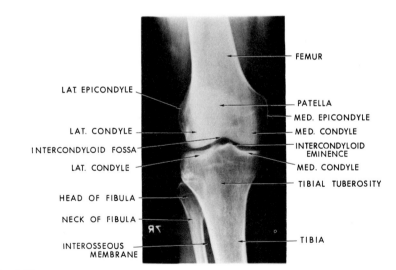

FEMUR

LAT. EPICONDYLE

PATELLA
MED. EPICONDYLE

LAT. CONDYLE
INTERCONDYLOID FOSSA
LAT. CONDYLE

MED. CONDYLE
INTERCONDYLOID EMINENCE
MED. CONDYLE

TIBIAL TUBEROSITY

HEAD OF FIBULA

NECK OF FIBULA

INTEROSSEOUS MEMBRANE

TIBIA

Fig. A-20.
Routine AP view of knee.

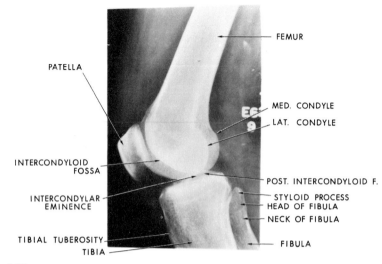

PATELLA

FEMUR

MED. CONDYLE

LAT. CONDYLE

INTERCONDYLOID
FOSSA

POST. INTERCONDYLOID F.

INTERCONDYLAR
EMINENCE

STYLOID PROCESS
HEAD OF FIBULA

NECK OF FIBULA

TIBIAL TUBEROSITY

TIBIA

FIBULA

Fig. A-21.

Routine lateral knee film.

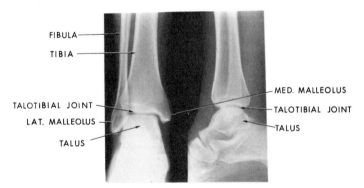

FIBULA

TIBIA

MED. MALLEOLUS

TALOTIBIAL JOINT

TALOTIBIAL JOINT

LAT. MALLEOLUS

TALUS

TALUS

Fig. A-22.

AP and lateral views of the ankle.

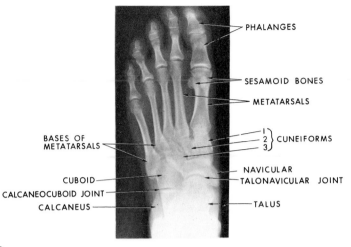

Fig. A-23.
Anteroposterior view of the foot.

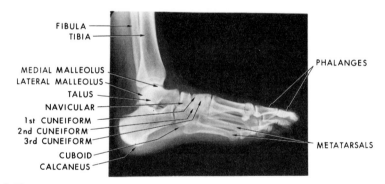

Fig. A-24.
Lateral view of the foot and ankle.

Index